Overcoming Migraine

Overcoming Migraine

A Comprehensive Guide to Treatment and Prevention by a Survivor

BETSY WYCKOFF

P•U•L•S•E

Station Hill Press

A P.U.L.S.E Book, published by Station Hill Press, Inc., Barrytown, New York 12507.

Distributed in the United States and Canada by The Talman Company, 150 Fifth Avenue, New York, New York 10011.

Cover art by Karen Poulson of Boulder, Colorado, who depicted her migraine pain in "Head Study" for the "Migraine Masterpieces" art competition sponsored by the National Headache Foundation and Wyeth-Ayerst Laboratories.

Library of Congress Cataloging-in-Publication Data
Wyckoff, Betsy.
    Overcoming Migraine : a comprehensive quide to treatment and prevention by a survivor / Betsy Wyckoff.
       p. cm.
    Includes bibliographical references.
    ISBN 0-88268-126-5 (cloth) : $21.95. — ISBN 0-88268-110-9 (pbk.)
: $9.95
    1. Migraine—Popular works. I. Title.
RC392.W93
616.8'57—dc20   90-23311
                                                    CIP

Acknowledgments

I would like to thank the National Headache Foundation in Chicago, the Migraine Foundation of Canada in Toronto, the Migraine Trust in London, and the Australian Bureau of Statistics for the migraine population figures in the Introduction. I would also like to thank the Migraine Trust for their help in the preparation of the list of headache clinics in the United Kingdom and Australia in Appendix III.

I would like to thank the National Headache Foundation and Wyeth-Ayerst Laboratories for permission to use the art from the "Migraine Masterpieces" exhibition. All of the art in this book was created by artists who are migraine sufferers.

Note to the Reader

Although the author has researched all sources thoroughly to ensure the accuracy of the information contained in this book, she assumes no responsibility for inaccuracies or omissions contained herein. Symptoms of, and tests for, the disorders discussed as well as drug dosages, side effects, precautions, interactions, and contra-indications should be confirmed by the reader in consultation with his or her personal physician.

Contents

This book is dedicated to my mother,
Pauline, who suffered in silence, and
to Julie for her support of my effort
to combat this disorder.

Introduction

Approximately 18 million people in the United States, over 4 million people in Canada, 5 million people in the United Kingdom, and almost 231 thousand people in Australia suffer from migraine headaches.[1] I am one of these people. I had intermittent migraines for twenty-five years before my daily migraines began. I experienced nausea and vomiting every day for three months and was finally diagnosed as having atypical migraine. This period was followed by five months of daily migraine headaches.

Life seemed hardly worth living. Eventually I became angry—angry at the pain, my doctors, and the side effects of the drugs I was taking. Mostly, I was angry at my own ignorance. I determined to research every bit of information existing on this condition. I read medical textbooks and journal articles as well as the more holistic fringe literature. All of the information I found is presented in this book. Because I believe people in pain do not have the patience to wade through a lengthy tome, I have organized my research findings as well as my own story into a concise presentation.

This book is the answer to the many questions I had about my migraines. I believe these are questions you, too, must have asked about your headaches.

First and foremost, I wondered if any migraine medications ex-

---

1. The Canadian figure includes people who have experienced one or more migraine attacks. Migraine need not be recurring for an individual to be counted. If U.K. and U.S.A. percentages are applied to the population of Australia, the number of migraine sufferers in that country rises to over 1 million.

isted whose side effects were not worse than the headache itself. I describe my search for these drugs in chapters 1 and 2. This material points out how horrendous the hunt for migraine medications can be if neither you nor your doctor knows very much about migraine treatment. The main purpose of these chapters is to help you become familiar with the various classes of migraine medications.

Next, I wondered if changes in my diet, environment, or lifestyle would help my headaches. Migraine triggers are discussed in chapters 3 and 4.

I thought my headaches might be a symptom of some other disease. The results of my search for disorders that can be accompanied by headache are outlined in chapter 5.

Since my headaches were worse during menstruation and menopause, I researched the connection between hormones and migraine. My findings are summarized in chapter 6.

At times I thought I had muscle contraction headaches and not migraines at all. I discuss the difference between these two kinds of headaches in chapter 7.

Biofeedback and other nonpharmacological treatments are explored in chapter 8.

Who are the experts in migraine management and how do you go about finding them? My answers to these questions are in chapter 9. The results of my inquiries into migraine prevention and treatment are summarized in chapter 10.

The dose, precautions, and side effects of various migraine medications are outlined in Appendix I. The physiology of migraine is discussed throughout the book. I pull all of this information into one place in Appendix II. Headache clinics in the United States, Canada, the United Kingdom, and Australia are listed in Appendix III. A list of migraine associations can be found in Appendix IV.

I believe I have touched upon everything that is known about migraine prevention and treatment. It is my firm belief that this book contains all the information needed to help you overcome this dreadful disorder. Be persistent. Have hope. A life free of pain is possible if you are willing to take action.

1

A Personal Migraine History

I first experienced migraine symptoms in my early twenties. I would get from two to three headaches every month, with one of these headaches coinciding with menstruation. Each headache would increase in severity throughout the day and would last approximately fourteen hours. The pain was located above my right eye and was throbbing in nature. My right nostril was stuffy and would run when the headache broke. At times the headache seemed to imitate a sinus infection. I had no nausea or vomiting, as is sometimes the case. I came to learn that what I had was labeled a "common" migraine, as opposed to the "classic" migraine in which there are visual symptoms, such as flashing lights, preceding the headache.

During one excruciating bout I went to my local hospital's emergency room where I was given Tylenol with codeine for the pain. The emergency room physician made appointments for me to have an electroencephalogram (EEG) and to see a neurologist. The EEG was negative. The neurologist told me my headache was caused by "nerves." I was so angry at being dismissed as just another neurotic female that I decided I would investigate headaches on my own. Fortunately, my local bookstore has a medical department with a well-stocked neurology section. In one of the textbooks I bought, I found a sentence stating that migraines could be caused by foods containing tyramine, a vasodilator. I was able to get a list of these foods, and when I stayed away from them, I had headaches only during menstruation.[1]

My headaches remained minimal until I reached menopause. During the first year of menopause I was free of headaches and I ate foods containing tyramine with fierce abandon. In January of my third year after starting menopause, I began a period of daily nausea and vomiting that lasted for three months.

My internist sent me for a series of tests, thinking a gall bladder ailment was the cause of my symptoms. The upper GI series and abdominal ultrasound revealed no disease. Since a brain tumor can cause nausea and vomiting, I had a brain scan using magnetic resonance imaging (MRI), which also revealed no tumor or other malady.

In the meantime, I had been taking a variety of antiemetic drugs. Of these, Compazine, Dramamine, Tigan, and Emetrol had little effect. Phenergan did seem to help the nausea to some extent, but I was unable to eat because of the nausea and lost almost 30 pounds in three months.

My internist referred me to a gastroenterologist who performed an endoscopic exam. This test was also negative. Because migraine runs in my family, the gastroenterologist diagnosed my symptoms as atypical migraine in which the nausea and vomiting masked an underlying migraine headache. He also felt I had status migrainosus in which one headache triggered the next, causing the symptoms to continue from day to day. I was given Torecan by this doctor. This antiemetic drug controlled the nausea more than any other medication I had tried.

Because my problem was now diagnosed as migraine, I returned to my internist to begin a series of treatments with traditional migraine medications. These treatments will be discussed in chapter 2.

In summary, over a period of twenty-five years, the frequency of my migraine headaches increased from approximately one a month to a three-month period of atypical migraine consisting of daily nausea and vomiting. Diagnosis was difficult and time-consuming because at this point I had no headache, only nausea.

---

1. These foods will be discussed in chapter 3.

2

Beginning Treatment

Such analgesics as aspirin, acetaminophen (Tylenol), and ibuprophen (Advil, Nuprin, Medipren) did little to alleviate my symptoms. Like aspirin and ibuprophen, Anaprox (naproxen) is an anti-inflammatory drug with analgesic properties. Many migraine sufferers find it to be an effective pain medication. Paradoxically, Anaprox intensified my symptoms.

The pain of migraine comes from vascular dilation. Ergotamine is used to treat migraine because of its vasoconstricting properties. The drug comes from a fungus that grows on rye. Ergotamine can be obtained in oral and sublingual tablets, in suppository form, as an aerosol, or can be administered by injection. Ergotamine should be taken at the very beginning of a migraine attack.

The side effects of ergotamine include nausea and, in cases where use is excessive, gangrene of the limbs. If taken for two days in a row, ergotamine may produce a rebound headache. Because the headache underlying my symptoms of nausea and vomiting was continual, my doctor prescribed Bellergal-S, which contains such a small amount of ergotamine it can be taken every day. Bellergal-S also contains phenobarbital, which is a sedative, as well as an ingredient to counteract the nausea caused by the ergotamine. The phenobarbital caused a paradoxical reaction in that it made me hyperactive. Bellergal-S, probably because of its low dose of ergotamine, did little to reverse my symptoms. However, for many people who only get migraines two or three times a month, ergotamine can be taken in a high enough dose to be an effective abortive agent.

The process that causes a headache is thought to begin with a period of vasoconstriction that is triggered by the release of serotonin, a neurotransmitter. As serotonin is absorbed, the amount is depleted. Lower serotonin levels produce vasodilation and headache. Since this process is triggered by the release of serotonin, any drug that regulates serotonin would be of value in migraine prevention. An antidepressant is just such a drug.

My doctor prescribed two antidepressants for me. Elavil (amitriptyline), the first, made me feel as if the skin were coming off my bones. The second antidepressant, Tofranil (imipramine), made me very jittery. Antidepressants were ruled out, and we next tried Fiorinal.

Fiorinal contains a barbiturate, aspirin, and caffeine. The sedative and muscle relaxant effects of Fiorinal are helpful in the treatment of tension headaches. Fiorinal did little to alleviate my migraine symptoms.

I was becoming desperate. My nausea was continuing, and no treatment was helping the migraine underlying the nausea. At this point I asked my internist to recommend a neurologist.

The first thing the neurologist did was to prescribe Reglan (metoclopramide) for my nausea. Nausea is often associated with a delay of gastric emptying, and thus prevents many migraine medications from being properly absorbed. Reglan relieves nausea and enhances the absorption of migraine medications because it increases gastric emptying. It has become the drug of choice in treating the nausea that may accompany migraine. Reglan can cause trembling as well as anxiety, but these side effects are usually transitory.

The neurologist's next major effort was to treat my atypical migraine, which had developed into a daily experience known as status migrainosus. By now I had had constant nausea and vomiting, but no headaches, for almost three months. The doctor prescribed prednisone, a steroid, for five days. Nothing happened. We waited for one week and tried the prednisone a second time. Again nothing happened. On the third course of prednisone my nausea disappeared and I began to experience the migraine that had been masked by the nausea. Daily migraine attacks were not aborted by additional prednisone.

In the meantime, I was treating the migraine with Tylenol and codeine. Although codeine is a narcotic, addiction to the drug is rare if it is not used on a daily basis. I was afraid of this drug and only used it when my symptoms became intolerable. I had previously used Tylenol and codeine for the nausea after the doctor convinced me that, even though I felt no pain, I should treat the nausea as a headache. He was right. The medication alleviated the nausea.

The beta blocking agents are used to treat heart problems as well as hypertension. Studies of patients with migraines revealed that some of these agents also prevent migraine attacks. Inderal (propranolol), Corgard (nadolol), Blocadren (timolol), Tenormin (atenolol), and Lopressor (metoprolol) are used in the treatment of migraine, with Inderal being the most effective of these agents. It is not known how beta blockers work to prevent migraine, but it is thought that one of their characteristics is to prevent the dilation of blood vessels.

The gastroenterologist, once he suspected migraine as the cause of my nausea, had prescribed Inderal for me. The drug stopped my symptoms, which confirmed his diagnosis of migraine. However, I could not tolerate the drug's side effects of breathlessness, fatigue, lethargy, and insomnia. The neurologist I was now seeing wanted me to try Corgard since we knew that at least one of the beta blocking class of drugs had worked for me. This drug penetrates the central nervous system poorly so it rarely causes insomnia. A trial run of Corgard proved to be ineffective in my case.

In spite of my experience, Inderal and the other beta blockers have proved to be some of the most powerful prophylatic agents used in migraine treatment. Inderal can be obtained in a sustained-released capsule that is administered once daily. It should be noted that patients with certain heart conditions, asthma, or diabetes cannot be treated with some of the beta blockers. Asthmatics and diabetics seem to react less strongly to Tenormin and Lopressor.

Sansert (methysergide) is another migraine medication that prevents headaches by inhibiting serotonin and constricting blood vessels. One of the many side effects of the drug is fibrosis or the forming of scar-like tissue in the heart and lungs. Sansert should be discontinued one month out of four to prevent this complication.

Although I have never taken LSD, Sansert (which is related to LSD) made me feel as if I was on a bad trip, with hallucinations being my major complaint. I was so frightened by my reaction to the drug that I went to a local hospital's emergency room for help. Before the emergency room staff got around to me, four hours had elapsed, and the effects of the drug had started to wear off. I left in disgust and swore to investigate the migraine medications I was taking with more diligence. As it turns out, I am one of the people that cannot tolerate Sansert. Although often a drug of last resort, Sansert has helped some migraine sufferers.

The calcium channel blockers dilate blood vessels. By blocking cellular calcium, they prevent the original constriction of the vessels by stopping the calcium needed for this reaction. As mentioned earlier, it is vasodilation in reaction to vasoconstriction that causes the head to ache.

My neurologist prescribed the calcium channel blocker Isoptin (verapamil) for me. I thought I was going to have a stroke on this drug. My head felt as if it were going to explode. The pressure was so intense I refused to continue using the drug. I could literally "feel" the vasodilating properties of Isoptin. I later learned that the calcium channel blockers are best taken when the cerebral arteries are in a state of rest, not after the headache has begun.

In spite of my experiences, these fairly new medications are considered by some headache specialists to hold much promise in the treatment of migraine. Other migraine specialists feel that the calcium channel blockers have been overrated in the prophylaxis of migraine because of their side effects and the long period needed before their effect is felt.

The doctor was beginning to understand that I react with great sensitivity to many migraine medications. Perhaps as a result, he next prescribed feverfew, a drug made from the dried leaves of a plant in the daisy family, *Tanacetum parthenium*. Feverfew can be obtained in most health food stores. It has anti-inflammatory properties and is thought to inhibit serotonin. In a very small percentage of users, feverfew's side effects include mouth ulcers, itchy skin, and a sore throat.

The leaves of the feverfew plant are freeze-dried and appear in capsule form. The usual dose is 125 mg once daily.[1] It is suggested that the herb not be used if you drink alcohol or are taking high blood pressure medicine. Painkillers retard the herb's effect, which may be why it did little to alter my headaches.

---

1. Hancock, K. (1986): *Feverfew: Your Headache May Be Over.* New Canaan, Connecticut : Keats Publishing.

Feverfew first became popular in England, and hundreds of migraine sufferers in that country testify to its value. It is especially appreciated because, unlike so many drugs used in migraine prevention, the side effects are minimal.

The neurologist told me his next plan was to give me anticonvulsive medication. Anticonvulsant drugs, such as Tegretol (carbamazepine) and Dilantin (phenytoin), have been used for many years to treat children with migraine, but the use of these drugs to treat adult migraine patients is controversial. Published studies using anticonvulsant drugs to treat migraine in nonepileptic adults are meager, although anecdotal reports do exist. Due to my previous experience with medications, the side effects of these drugs made me very wary. I felt my doctor was grasping at straws. Before taking any more drugs, I decided it was time to get another opinion. By now my headaches had continued on a daily basis, in one form or another, for over eight months.

I first went to the headache clinic at the Montefiore Medical Center in Bronx, New York. After an extensive examination, the neurologist suggested I try Inderal, Anaprox, and Midrin. He felt I should use Inderal as an abortive agent in which I would take only the morning dose, and in this way I might avoid the side effects that accompanied Inderal in the past. Inderal taken in this fashion has, at times, bought me up to eight hours of headache relief.

Anaprox used on a daily basis has been found to prevent headaches. However, I was one of the 5 percent of the people in whom the drug produced headaches.

Midrin contains isometheptene mucate (a vasoconstrictor), dichloralphenazone (a mild sedative), and acetaminophen (an analgesic). It is a good abortive agent for mild to moderate migraine. Midrin is similar to ergotamine in its actions but has less severe side effects. For example, Midrin does not cause nausea. It also does not produce rebound headaches. The usual dose is 2 capsules to start.[1] These may be followed by 1 capsule every hour up to 5 per day.[2] Do not exceed 15 capsules per week.[3] I found Midrin to be one of the more successful drugs that had been prescribed for my migraines.

---

1. Diamond, S. and Millstein, E. (1988): Current concepts of migraine therapy. *Journal of Clinical Pharmacology.* 28: 195.
2. Ibid.
3. Ibid.

My next step was to call the National Headache Foundation in Chicago to request their physician membership list for my area. The number in Illinois is 1-800-523-8858; outside of Illinois the number is 1-800-843-2256. I felt that any neurologist who belonged to the foundation would be particularly interested in headaches.

The next neurologist that I saw prescribed lithium for me. Lithium is used for chronic cluster headaches. Its use for migraine is controversial. People on lithium must be closely supervised. A high blood level can cause shakiness or confusion. Long-time use can cause kidney and thyroid problems. In some cases, lithium makes migraine worse. On the other hand, lithium seems to help people with cyclic migraine in whom headaches occur daily for six weeks or so and then stop for several weeks. Because this was not the pattern of my headaches, I decided to put lithium on hold for a while.

After reviewing all of the drugs used in migraine treatment, I realized I had not explored the tricyclic antidepressants thoroughly. I knew that although I could not tolerate Elavil or Tofranil, that did not mean I would have the same experience with other drugs in this class. Aventyl (nortriptyline) and Sinequan (doxepin) are two of several antidepressants reported to prevent migraine headaches. Sinequan and Tofranil inhibit both serotonin and norepinephrine, Aventyl mainly inhibits norepinephrine, and Elavil acts primarily as an inhibitor of serotonin.

Sinequan has turned out to be a good migraine prophylactic medication for me. Because it can cause drowsiness, Sinequan is taken once a day at bedtime. I have a reverse reaction in that instead of drowsiness, as little as 10 milligrams can cause increased energy levels and insomnia. For this reason, I take Sinequan in the morning. I now believe if I had taken only 10 milligrams of Elavil instead of 25 milligrams, I might have found headache relief months earlier.

Catapres (clonidine) is one drug used in the treatment of migraine that I have not tried. It is normally used to treat high blood pressure. Catapres should be discontinued slowly to prevent hypertension. The side effects of this drug include dry mouth, drowsiness, and dizziness. It has been found to be disappointing in migraine treatment. In some studies it was no more effective than a placebo.

Periactin (cyproheptadine) blocks histamine and serotonin receptors. It is primarily used to treat migraine in children but has been helpful in some cases of adult migraine. I have not used this drug because I have a paradoxical reaction to antihistamines in that they cause headaches rather than prevent them. Periactin cannot be combined with alcohol or MAO inhibitors. It can cause seizures in epileptics. Its side effects in adults include sedation, weight gain, dizziness, and dry mouth.

Caffeine has been known to abort migraine headaches because of its vasoconstricting properties. One migraine sufferer swears that a NoDoz tablet every morning prevents her daily migraines. Too much caffeine, however, can cause a rebound headache.

Dihydroergotamine (DHE) nasal spray and pizotifen are two migraine medications not available in the United States. DHE nasal spray has shown promise in aborting the occasional migraine. DHE nasal spray is rapidly absorbed and has fewer side effects than other ergotamine preparations. Pizotifen is a preventative migraine medication. Although the drug helps some people, not all migraine sufferers who take pizotifen find it effective. The drug's side effects include increased appetite and drowsiness.

Glaxo Inc. has a new drug, GR43175 (Sumatriptan), that reportedly aborts migraines without the side effects of ergotamine. The drug, now in clinical trials, is not expected to be on the market for several years.

Each migraine sufferer reacts to the drugs discussed in this chapter differently. In my case I have found Midrin to be helpful in aborting a migraine once it has begun. Midrin is a vasoconstrictor. If the headache is not completely aborted, I take one Tylenol with codeine in addition to Midrin. Abortive medications are listed in Table 2.1.

Table 2.1
Abortive Medications

MEDICATION	INGREDIENTS	COMMENTS
Analgesics		
Aspirin	Acetylsalicylic acid 227-400 mg. (May be combined with acetaminophen, caffeine, or buffers)	Overuse may cause internal bleeding. Buffers reduce stomach irritation

MEDICATION	INGREDIENTS	COMMENTS
Advil, Nuprin, Medipren	Ibuprophen 200 mg	More than 1000 mg per day of aspirin or Tylenol can cause rebound headaches
Tylenol	Acetaminophen 325 or 500 mg	
Tylenol with codeine	Acetaminophen 300 mg, codeine phosphate 7.5, 15, 30 and 60 mg	Can cause habituation

Nonsteroidal anti-inflammatory

Anaprox	Naproxen sodium 275 mg	Take with food or antacid to prevent nausea

Ergotamine

Cafergot (oral)	Ergotamine tartrate 1 mg, caffeine 100 mg.	Continual use can cause rebound headaches. Do not exceed 6 tablets per day or 10 tablets per week of oral dose.[1] Do not exceed 2 suppositories per day or 5 suppositories per week of rectal dose.[2]
Cafergot (rectal)	Ergotamine tartrate 2 mg, caffeine 100 mg	
Wigraine (oral)	Ergotamine tartrate 1 mg, caffeine 100 mg	
Wigraine (rectal)	Ergotamine tartrate 2 mg, caffeine 100 mg	
Medihaler Ergotamine (aerosol)	Ergotamine tartrate. One dose contains 0.36 mg	One dose every 5 minutes.[3] Do not exceed 6 doses per day or 10 doses per week[4]

1. Diamond, S. and Millstein, E. (1988): Current concepts of migraine therapy. *Journal of Clinical Pharmacology.* 28: 195.
2. Ibid.
3. Ibid.
4. Ibid

MEDICATION	INGREDIENTS	COMMENTS
Ergomar, Ergostat (sublingual)	Ergotamine tartrate 2 mg	One tablet at onset to be repeated every 30 minutes.[1] Do not exceed 3 per day or 5 per week[2]
Midrin	Isometheptene mucate 65 mg, dichloralphenazone 100 mg, acetaminophen 325 mg	Take 2 capsules at onset followed by 1 capsule every hour up to 5.[3] Do not exceed 5 capsules per day or 15 per week[4]
Beta blocker		
Inderal	Propranolol 10, 20, 40, 60, or 80 mg	As little as 10 mg may abort headache
Antiemetic		
Reglan	Metoclopramide 10 mg	
NoDoz	Caffeine 100 mg	Caffeine is a vasoconstrictor. More than 2 tablets may cause a rebound headache. Do not exceed limit by combining with other medications or drinks containing caffeine

Prophylactic drugs are appropriate for people who get more than one or two migraines each week. These medications are taken daily to prevent a headache from even beginning. I have found the anti-depressant drug Sinequan to be effective in eliminating my migraine headaches. The more common prophylactic drugs used in the treatment of migraine are listed in Table 2.2.

1. Ibid.
2. Ibid.
3. Ibid
4. Ibid

In summary, throughout the course of three months of nausea and five months of daily migraine, I became a test subject for various migraine medications. To be well informed before starting treatment study the drugs listed in Table 2.1 and Table 2.2.

The drugs listed in Table 2.1 will stop a migraine attack once it has started. There are five major drug groups in this category: analgesics, anti-inflammatories, ergotamine compounds, Midrin, and the beta blockers. The prophylactic drugs listed in Table 2.2 are taken daily to prevent headaches from arising. They are appropriate if you get migraines on a weekly basis. The five most effective groups of drugs in this category are: the beta blockers, anti-inflammatory drugs, antidepressants, Sansert and the calcium channel blockers.

Table 2.2
Prophylactic Medications

MEDICATION	INGREDIENTS	COMMENTS
Beta blockers		
Inderal	Propranolol hydrochloride 10, 20, 40, 60, 80 mg	Inderal is the most effective of the beta blockers
Corgard	Nadolol 40, 80, 120, 160 mg	Insulin-using diabetics and asthmatics do better on Tenormin or Lopressor
Lopressor	Metoprolol tartrate 50, 100 mg	
Blocadren	Timolol maleate 10, 20 mg	
Tenormin	Atenolol 50, 100 mg	Corgard and Tenormin produce less insomnia

MEDICATION	INGREDIENTS	COMMENTS

Ergotamine

Bellergal	Ergotamine tartrate 0.3 mg, phenobarbital 20 mg, belladonna 0.1 mg	
Bellergal-S	Ergotamine tartrate 0.6 mg, phenobarbital 40 mg, belladonna 0.2 mg	

Nonsteroidal anti-inflammatories

Anaprox	Naproxen sodium 275 mg	Take with food or antacid to prevent nausea
Naprosyn	Naproxen 250, 375, 500 mg	

Antidepressants

Elavil	Amitriptyline hydrochloride 10, 25, 50, 75, 100, 150 mg	
Aventyl	Nortriptyline hydrochloride 10, 25, 50, 75 mg	
Sinequan	Doxepin hydrochloride 10, 25, 50, 75, 100, 150 mg	
Nardil	Phenelzine sulfate 15 mg	MAO inhibitor. Avoid foods containing tyramine

MEDICATION	INGREDIENTS	COMMENTS
Sansert	Methysergide maleate 2 mg	Must be stopped after 4 months to prevent fibrosis. Side effects are common
Calcium channel blockers		
Isoptin	Verapamil hydrochloride 80, 120 mg	Vasodilators
Procardia	Nifedipine 10 mg	
Periactin	Cyproheptadine hydrochloride 4 mg	Antihistamine. Used in treating childhood migraine
Feverfew	*Tanacetum parthenium* 125 mg	Do not take with high dosage high blood pressure medicine or alcohol. Herb. Obtain in health food stores. Dosage is 125 mg per day [1]

---

1. Hancock, K. (1986): *Feverfew: Your Headache May Be Over*. New Canaan, Connecticut: Keats Publishing.

3

Diet and Migraine

People subject to migraines often do not metabolize amines properly. They seem to lack the enzyme necessary to break down these substances. Amines influence the diameter of the blood vessels. Dilated blood vessels produce the pain we know as headache. Tyramine (cheese), phenylethylamine (chocolate), and octopamine (citrus) are examples of the amines in our diet that may trigger a headache.

Nitrites are used as a food preservative. They also trigger headaches in some people, and foods containing this chemical should be avoided. Nitrites may be found in hot dogs, bacon, ham, salami, bologna, sausage, pepperoni, and many other packaged meats.

Foods containing the sugar substitute aspartame are known to produce headaches. Saccharin, on the other hand, is not a migraine trigger. Monosodium glutamate (MSG) is used to enhance the flavor of instant rice, soups, and Chinese food. MSG will precipitate a headache in many people.

Although not listed in the literature as a migraine precipitant, I have found the preservative sodium benzoate to be a migraine trigger.

Reading food labels is extremely important. For example, I was surprised when I got a migraine after eating a cream cheese-smoked salmon dip, since cream cheese is one of the few cheeses that does not contain tyramine. I then read the label on the package only to discover that this product contains MSG. The morning after eating a dinner of steak, rice, and salad, I awoke with a pounding migraine. I read the label on the steak sauce and salad dressing that I had had the night before to discover that both contained the preservative sodium benzoate, a powerful migraine trigger in my case. I could have avoided this headache if I had been in the habit of reading food labels.

Foods containing amines, nitrites, aspartame, MSG, or sodium benzoate should be avoided by many people prone to headaches. These foods are listed in Table 3.1.

Table 3.1

Foods Containing Amines and Other Substances Known to Trigger Headaches

Fruits

Citrus	Avocados
Bananas	Papaya
Canned figs	Pineapples
Dates	Red plums
Raisins	Raspberries
Strawberries	Mangoes

Vegetables

Spinach	Italian broad beans
Lima beans	Pea pods
Soybeans	Sauerkraut
Onions	Fava beans
Garbanzo beans	Lentils
Olives	Snow peas
Pinto beans	Pickles
Navy beans	Tomato
Eggplant	

Meats

Turkey	Game meats
Liver, sweetbreads, kidneys, brains	Salted or smoked fish (lox, anchovies)

Pickled herring

Pork

Preserved meat

Caviar

Chicken livers, pâté

Milk products

Cream

Yogurt

Cheese (except cream cheese
and cottage cheese)

Sour cream

Buttermilk

Chocolate

Alcohol

Beer

Sherry

Red wine

Yeast

Fresh coffee cake

Homemade breads

Brewer's yeast

Doughnuts

Sourdough breads

Vinegar (except white vinegar) found in:

Relishes

Catsup

Mustard

Salad dressing

Worcestershire sauce

Steak sauce

Chili sauce

Nuts and peanut butter

Potatoes

Seeds

Sunflower

Pumpkin

Sesame

Coffee

Nitrites found in:

Hot dogs

Bologna

Bacon	Sausage
Ham	Pepperoni
Salami	

Sugar substitute
Aspartame

Monosodium glutamate (MSG) found in:

Chinese foods	Dry roasted nuts
Instant rice	Instant gravies
Soup	Potato chips
TV dinners	Meat tenderizers and seasonings

Miscellaneous

Soy products (bean curd, miso soup)	Sodium benzoate
Licorice	Garlic

In addition to the foods presented in Table 3.1, peas, milk, wheat, eggs, corn, fish, tea, apples, and cabbage have been reported to trigger headaches in a minority of people. These foods, which are listed in Table 3.2, do not contain nitrates, MSG, or such amines as tyramine, phenylethylamine, or octopamine. Their manner of provoking headaches is not known.

Table 3.2
Nonamine Food Triggers

Peas	Corn
Fish	Milk
Tea	Wheat
Apples	Eggs
Cabbage	

Such alcoholic beverages as red wine, beer, and sherry trigger headaches. Alcoholic beverages less likely to provoke a headache include white wine, rum, scotch, and vodka. The kind of headache I am referring to is a migraine resulting from serotonin-provoked vasodilation and should not be confused with the hangover headache that results several hours after drinking has stopped. The hangover headache is a withdrawal symptom and has nothing to do with migraine. It happens to anyone who has consumed too much alcohol.

Coffee, because of its amine content, can trigger a headache. The caffeine in coffee is also a headache trigger. More than two cups of coffee may produce caffeine withdrawal symptoms that include a headache. It would be wise not to exceed 200 mg of caffeine daily. This amount includes the caffeine in coffee, tea, soda, and in such medications as aspirin and various ergot preparations. The median amount of caffeine in coffee and tea is listed in Table 3.3.

Table 3.3

Caffeine Content of Coffee and Tea

Brewed coffee/cup	100 mg[1]
Instant coffee/cup	85 mg
Tea/cup	70 mg

If you decide to give up coffee and tea altogether, do so gradually. I experienced one of my worse migraines when I stopped my consumption of coffee abruptly.

Add up the caffeine in the coffee and tea you drink each day. Add to this figure the caffeine in any medications you might be taking (see Tables 2.1 and 2.2), the caffeine in the aspirin you take (which is listed on the label), and the caffeine in your soft drinks. The total amount might surprise you.

Serotonin is an amine made in the body from dietary tryptophan. Turkey contains tryptophan. As we learned earlier, altered serotonin levels can trigger vasodilation and headache. I have found turkey, because of its relationship to serotonin, to be a migraine trigger.

The preservative benzoic acid and the yellow dye tartrazine (FD & C No. 5) have been reported to cause headaches in some people. Children seem especially susceptible to these food additives. Sodium benzoate, which I have found to be a migraine trigger, is the sodium salt of benzoic acid.

---

1. These figures represent an average.

Low blood sugar can cause migraine headaches because this condition starts a chemical chain reaction that results in dilated cerebral blood vessels. In some people, refined sugar stimulates the pancreas to release excess insulin that metabolizes not only the sugar just eaten but also any sugar already present in the bloodstream. The result is a lower blood sugar level than before the sugar was eaten. By avoiding sugar altogether, this process of rapid rise/rapid fall in blood sugar levels does not take place, thus preventing a migraine from developing.

Sugar that should be avoided includes sucrose, glucose (dextrose), fructose, maltose, and corn syrup. Food labels must be read. The most unsuspecting foods often contain sugar, and even a very small amount can trigger a headache in some people.

If all refined sugar is avoided, where does the body get its energy? The natural sugar in fresh fruit and unsweetened fruit juice does not trigger the insulin chain reaction outlined above. Another source is such carbohydrates as rice, bread, and pasta. Some carbohydrates should be eaten with each meal to offset the lack of refined sugar in your diet.

The sugar level in the blood also decreases when too much time has elapsed between meals. Some migraine sufferers have found that if they eat every four hours, their headaches disappear. A protein snack at bedtime will often prevent a morning headache. I have found, for example, that I can eliminate morning migraines by having a sandwich before going to bed.

If your blood sugar is abnormally low, you might have a condition called hypoglycemia. Your doctor can determine if you are hypoglycemic by giving you a glucose tolerance test. Symptoms of hypoglycemia include lightheadedness, sweating, and headache. Even if you are not hypoglycemic, headache can result if you do not have something to eat every four hours. Many migraine sufferers have had their headaches totally stop when they ate every four hours, had a protein snack at bedtime, and stopped eating refined sugar.

I avoid all of the amine-containing foods listed in Table 3.1. The few times I have cheated and eaten one of these foods, a headache has usually followed. I was able to see what other foods might trigger a headache by eliminating all foods for up to five days except those with no headache causing potential (Table 3.3). At the end of this period, I reintroduced foods one at a time to my diet. If a headache developed, I knew that food would have to be eliminated. I also ate bedtime and between meal snacks from Table 3.3 so that no more than four hours would elapse without some food intake during waking hours. Headaches may get worse before improving during this testing period.

Table 3.3

Foods With No Known Headache Causing Potential

Meat

Lamb	Chicken

Fruit

Pears	Unsweetened pear juice

Vegetables

Brussels sprouts	Carrots
Zucchini	Broccoli
Cauliflower	

After adding back a fair amount of foods, I found that eggs, wheat, and milk were all headache triggers for me. When I avoided these foods, amine-containing foods, nitrites, MSG, sodium benzoate, and the sugar substitute aspartame, my headaches decreased considerably. For the first time in eight months, I had headache-free periods that lasted for days.

In summary, many migraine sufferers have to accept the fact that they cannot eat foods containing amines if they want to become headache free. It should be noted that upon occasion a small amount of amine-containing foods can be tolerated; but once we go over a certain critical level, headache results. Since we cannot always predict what this level is, it is best to avoid these foods altogether. In addition, sugar should be eliminated from the diet for at least a month to see if you find relief. Do not skip meals. The foods you eat are powerful migraine triggers, and many headaches can be avoided by alterations in the diet.

4

Nondietary Migraine Triggers

In addition to diet, migraine triggers include stress, sleep, altitude, chemicals, medicines, vitamins, weather, flickering light, exercise, and sex.

Research has shown that migraineurs are not more sensitive to stress than nonmigraineurs. Some migraine authorities suggest that stress releases serotonin. It is the reaction to serotonin, and not a particular susceptibility to stress, that causes the headache. Some migraineurs get their headaches during the let down period following the stressful situation when serotonin levels are falling.

Discussing stress as a migraine trigger is a complicated issue because it implies that migraine sufferers are overly sensitive people who cannot handle stress properly. This is simply not the case. Until approximately ten years ago, migraine sufferers were thought to be obsessive, perfectionist, driven people. Personality tests given since that time show that the personality traits of migraineurs do not differ from those of the general population. Migraine sufferers do not have unique personalities that would predispose them to be particularly sensitive to stress. I prefer to think of migraineurs as people in whom stress sets up a biochemical alteration that produces headache. It is this constitutional biochemical process, and not environmental stress per se, that triggers the migraine attack.

Excessive or too little sleep may also precipitate a migraine. Sleeping late over the weekend is a common cause of headaches. It is best to get up at the same time each day, including weekends.

Vasodilation at altitudes above 8000 feet, brought about by a reduction in oxygen, can cause headaches. I remember camping in the Sierra Nevada mountains many years ago. I was feeling fine until I had a glass of red wine while sitting around the campfire. The combination of the two triggers—altitude and red wine—resulted in a terrible migraine.

A variety of chemicals, including carbon tetrachloride, benzene, insecticides, and home insulation products made from formaldehyde, have been reported to cause headaches. Strong smells, a smoke-filled room, or a poorly ventilated room may trigger a headache. Carbon monoxide can be a migraine trigger. Some people report less frequent and less intense headaches when they stop smoking. This may be because carbon monoxide is present in cigarette smoke. Smokers have been found to have a higher blood level of carbon monoxide than nonsmokers.

Some medicines can trigger a migraine. Nitroglycerin is used to treat heart disease and has been known to cause migraines. Other migraine triggers include lithium, the antihypertensive drugs reserpine and hydralazine, the anti-inflammatory drug indomethacin, diuretics, and the bronchodilating drug Aminophylline and the other theophyllines. If you get migraines and are taking any of these drugs, you should ask your doctor to change your prescription.

Sinus and cold medications may trigger headaches. I would be wary of any compounds containing ephedrine (a decongestant), chlorpheniramine maleate (an antihistamine), or phenylpropanolamine (a decongestant). A chemical that has "amine" as part of its name should be avoided. I recently bought a cold medication that promised relief without drowsiness. Not containing antihistamines, I thought this drug would be safe. The next morning I had a cold that was now accompanied by a migraine. I read the label only to discover this medication contained the migraine trigger ephedrine.

Withdrawal headaches from aspirin, acetaminophen, and ergotamine occur with daily use of these drugs. More of the drug is then taken to combat the withdrawal headache. A cycle is established that leads to chronic daily headaches and dependence on these drugs to relieve the headache that they have caused. More than 1000 mg of aspirin or acetaminophen must be taken daily in order for withdrawal headaches to occur.

A chronic headache sufferer can easily exceed 1000 mg of aspirin or acetaminophen each day. For example, in order to combat a particularly bad migraine, I had taken three Tylenol tablets and two Midrin capsules in the course of one day for a total of 1625 mg of acetaminophen. A withdrawal headache followed, which I could have treated with more Tylenol and Midrin. If I had done so, my headache would have become chronic, and dependency on these drugs would have ensued.

Some migraine patients do not even think of aspirin or Tylenol as drugs. They take them much as they might take vitamins. Taking two or three aspirin or Tylenol each morning might have become a life-long habit. According to some migraine authorities, daily headaches are withdrawal symptoms from the chronic use of ergotamine, aspirin, or acetaminophen. Stopping such chronic use is very hard and may require hospitalization. One way to break the habit is to taper off of these drugs by taking less each day. Another way is to stop their use abruptly. You may experience a headache for from three to seven days before the headache disappears entirely. If you have stopped all of the triggers listed in this book and your headache continues on a daily basis, chances are it is caused by one or more of the medications you are taking.

Antianxiety drugs, such as Librium and Valium, serve no purpose in the treatment of migraine. Even a small amount of these drugs can cause withdrawal headaches. If your doctor has prescribed an antianxiety drug for your migraines, please get a second opinion about your need for this medication.

Even vitamin pills are not as benign as we once thought. From 25,000 to 50,000 IU of vitamin A may trigger a headache. If you eat foods that are high in vitamin A, such as carrots, and take a supplement with 25,000 IU of A, you would be over your limit, and a headache could result. Large doses of niacin (nicotinic acid) can also trigger a migraine. Nicotinic acid is a vasodilator and should only be taken during the aura phase in classic migraine.

Many vitamins contain such migraine triggers as yeast, citrus, and soy. If you must take vitamins, you might want to take one of the hypo-allergenic brands that avoid these substances. I have found many vitamin pills to be migraine triggers.

I have also found that one 600 mg tablet of calcium is safe, while two 600 mg tablets of calcium per day will trigger a headache. It is not the calcium, but rather the other ingredients that the manufacturers put in the pills that are the headache triggers. At the present time, I am experimenting with calcium made from oyster shells, since it is a pure substance with no added ingredients.

Weather conditions can precipitate a migraine attack. Wind, a thunderstorm, the sun's glare on snow or water, and very cold temperatures or high humidity are migraine triggers for some people. I am particularly sensitive to strong sunlight on a hot day. If I do not wear a hat and sunglasses at the beach, the heat and glare of the sun will trigger a headache.

Some people find that the flickering light from a television or movie screen or the flicker from fluorescent lights will trigger a headache. Wearing sunglasses or tinted lenses may help this condition.

Exercise can also be a migraine trigger, especially vigorous exercise by people not physically fit. Exercise headaches can reflect a serious medical problem. You should see your doctor if you get headaches while exercising.

The orgasmic headache, most common in men, is a form of effort headache that occurs during orgasm. Like the exercise headache, orgasmic headaches may indicate a serious underlying condition and should be discussed with your doctor.

Nondietary migraine triggers are listed in Table 4.1.

Table 4.1

Nondietary Migraine Triggers

Stress

Sleep

| Excessive | Fatigue |

Altitude

Chemicals

Carbon tetrachloride	Benzene
Insecticides	Formaldehyde
Carbon monoxide	

Environment

| Strong smells | Smoke |
| Poor ventilation | Flickering light |

Medicines

Nitroglycerin	Hydralazine
Lithium	Reserpine
Indomethacin	Diuretics
Antihistamines	Aspirin
Acetaminophen	Ergotamine
Librium, Valium	Decongestants with
Theophyllines	phenylpropanolamine or
(Aminophylline)	ephedrine

Vitamins

Vitamin A	Niacin

Weather

Wind	Thunderstorms
Glare	Cold temperatures
High humidity	

Exercise

Sex

In summary, a variety of environmental conditions and nondietary substances can trigger a migraine. I would suggest paying particular attention to your sleep patterns. Try not to get too much or too little sleep. Also, to avoid withdrawal headaches, take less than 1000 mg of aspirin or Tylenol daily and do not use ergotamine medications every day.

5

Headache as a Symptom of Disease

A basic question must be asked about any migraine headache. Is it a disease in and of itself, or is it a symptom of an underlying disorder? This question is especially important if migraine attacks have just begun or if ongoing migraines change in their frequency, intensity, or characteristics. The computed axiel tomography (CAT) scan or magnetic resonance imaging (MRI) and blood tests are routinely given to determine the cause of the headache. Depending on symptoms, an angiogram, lumbar puncture, or other tests might also be called for.

A brain tumor is something that all headache patients fear. A CAT scan or MRI takes X-ray type pictures of the brain that show the presence of a tumor. Brain tumors are very rare but their possibility must be ruled out immediately.

Sixty percent of the people who have brain tumors will have a headache. In the majority of these cases, the pain is dull, nonthrobbing, and intermittent. It may be made worse by changing positions or coughing. The headache may be accompanied by loss of smell or hearing, personality changes, alterations in vision, loss of balance, and weakness or numbness in one-half of the body. Approximately 50 percent of people with brain tumors experience nausea and vomiting.

A hemorrhage from a ruptured aneurysm produces a violent, continuous headache, which may be accompanied by vomiting, a stiff neck, drowsiness, and loss of consciousness. The headache comes suddenly and is sometimes described as feeling like an explosion. A CAT scan or MRI will reveal a ruptured aneurysm. An unruptured aneurysm may also be signaled by a headache described as similar to an explosion or a clap of thunder. An angiogram is used to locate the unruptured aneurysm.

Infections are a common cause of headache. The presence of many infections can be determined by blood tests.

Daily headache may be one of the symptoms of the Epstein-Barr virus. Other symptoms include malaise, fatigue, lymph node enlargement, fever, and a sore throat. In some cases, headache and fatigue continue after other symptoms cease to exist.

Lyme disease is an infection transmitted by mouse or deer ticks. In addition to headache, Lyme disease may produce malaise, fatigue, arthritis-like symptoms, stiff neck, muscular pain, and fever. If untreated, neurological abnormalities may develop.

Meningitis is an infection that causes headache, fever, neck stiffness, seizures, vomiting, and an aversion to bright light. It is an inflammation of the covering of the brain, the meninges, which is usually produced by a viral or bacterial infection.

Unlike viral meningitis, bacterial meningitis can be life-threatening. The infecting agent gains entry into the brain through the nose, sinuses, ear, or bloodstream. The diagnosis of meningitis can be confirmed by an examination of spinal fluid that is removed by lumbar puncture.

Other infections accompanied by headache include tonsillitis, pneumonia, scarlet fever, typhoid fever, typhus fever, influenza, smallpox, rabies, mumps, measles, herpes simplex, poliomyelitis, and malaria. In most cases, the headache disappears when the infection subsides.

Multiple sclerosis is another serious disease that is accompanied by head pain in a minority of cases. MRI and spinal fluid examination are good diagnostic indicators of this disease. Symptoms of multiple sclerosis may include spasticity, tremor, disturbances of speech, ocular movements, impaired vision, bladder problems, and weakness, numbness, or paralysis in one or more extremity.

The mouth and eyes can also be the source of headaches. Abscesses in the mouth and cracked teeth can lead to head pain that may resemble migraine. If you have headaches, a checkup by your dentist is in order.

Eye strain as well as a rare form of glaucoma can cause headaches. An eye examination by an ophthalmologist will disclose the presence of these conditions.

Systemic lupus erythematosus, giant cell arteritis (or temporal arteritis, as it is sometimes called), and polymyalgia rheumatica are three inflammatory diseases that often include headache as one of their symptoms.

Lupus is a disease that damages the connective tissue throughout the body. Inflammation of the membranes surrounding the kidneys, lungs, joints, and other organs is common. In addition to headaches, a few of the many symptoms of lupus are fever, muscle pain, fatigue, anemia, weight loss, joint pain, hair loss, and sometimes a red rash on the face and other areas exposed to the sun. Blood tests will confirm a diagnosis of lupus.

Giant cell arteritis is an inflammatory disease of the arteries of the temples that usually develops in people over 50 years of age. The headache that accompanies this disorder is a dull ache that may be sharp at times on one or both sides of the head. The pain is described as having a burning quality. There may be tenderness or swelling of the temporal artery. The pain itself may radiate to this artery. The headache is often slightly worse at night. Muscular aches and pains, weight loss, low-grade fever, fatigue, scalp tenderness, and jaw claudication, or pain when chewing, are symptomatic of the disease. If not treated, giant cell arteritis can lead to blindness and stroke. Blood tests may show an elevated sedimentation rate, abnormal liver function, and anemia. The diagnosis of giant cell arteritis can be confirmed by a biopsy of the temporal artery.

Polymyalgia rheumatica is caused by an inflammation of the muscles. It is characterized by muscle aches in the neck, shoulders, and hips. It usually does not affect people under 50 years of age. Other symptoms include headache, morning stiffness, fatigue, weight loss and a low-grade fever. Some people think polymyalgia rheumatica and giant cell arteritis represent different stages in the same disease process. Blood test abnormalities are similar in both diseases.

Many people who have a heart malfunction known as mitral valve prolapse also suffer from headaches. Other symptoms of this condition include fatigue, chest pain, palpitations, and dizziness. Platelet aggregation on the abnormal valve may play a role in the development of headache. Echocardiography is used to confirm the diagnosis of mitral valve prolapse.

Cushing's syndrome is a disorder resulting from increased production of cortisol by the adrenal gland. Elevated cortisol levels can
be caused by an adrenal tumor, a pituitary tumor, or prolonged use
of steroid medications. Approximately one-half of the patients with
this syndrome experience headaches. In addition, fatigue, muscle
weakness, osteoporosis, obesity, hypertension, a "moon face," and,
in women, cessation of menses and excessive face and body hair are
common symptoms of the disease. The diagnosis of Cushing's syndrome is based on the results of a dexamethasone-suppression test.

Anywhere from 30 to 80 percent of head injury patients experience headaches. The headache that results from a concussion may
be either dull or throbbing in nature. Movement of the head or body
may worsen the headache. It may be accompanied by amnesia,
irritability, nausea, vomiting, vertigo, or difficulty in concentration.
The headache may develop days or weeks after the injury and can
last from days to years. Headache also commonly follows whiplash
injuries, along with vertigo, dizziness, ringing in the ears, and visual
disturbances. In addition, some people experience mood changes,
anxiety, difficulties in thinking, and insomnia following an injury to
the head. X-rays may be required after a concussion to detect a
possible fracture. A CAT scan might be necessary to rule out hemorrhage following a severe blow to the head.

Common disorders accompanied by headache, along with their
diagnostic tests, are listed in Table 5.1. Uncommon causes of headaches include very high blood pressure, cervical spine disease, a jaw
disorder called temporomandibular joint (TMJ) dysfunction, constipation, and sinus disease.

The headache caused by high blood pressure is usually experienced as pain in the back of the head and neck. The blood pressure
must be severely elevated in order to produce head pain. In some
cases, it is the medication used to treat high blood pressure that is
the cause of the headache.

In cervical spine disease, rheumatoid arthritis and nerve root
entrapment due to osteoarthritic changes in the cervical spine can
cause pain in the neck and back of the head that sometimes radiates
to the forehead. Most of the neck pain experienced by headache
sufferers, however, stems from conditions other than cervical spine
disease. The majority of people with rheumatoid arthritis or degen-
erative diseases of the spine do not have chronic headaches.

Head pain from TMJ dysfunction originates in the jaw and can
radiate to the ear and temple. A click in the jaw when chewing or

talking may indicate the presence of this condition. The pain is thought to be due to muscle spasms resulting from grinding or clenching the teeth or from an uneven bite. Many professionals feel that the connection between TMJ dysfunction and headache has been exaggerated.

Headache resulting from constipation is a controversial issue. Some experts feel that accumulated toxins or an expanded bowel can precipitate a headache. Other authorities see no connection between headache and constipation.

You might wonder why sinus disease is listed as an "uncommon" cause of headaches. Pain results when the sinuses become filled with fluid as a result of infection, tumors, or allergic reactions. These conditions are rare and many so-called sinus headaches are in reality muscle contraction or migraine headaches. X-rays will indicate the presence of sinus disease.

The removal of spinal fluid during lumbar puncture may cause a headache of short duration. Lying down and drinking fluids helps relieve the headache. As soon as spinal fluid pressure returns to normal, the pain disappears.

Table 5.1

Common Disorders Accompanied by Headache

DISORDER	TEST
Brain tumor	MRI or CAT scan
Aneurysm	
Ruptured	MRI or CAT scan
Unruptured	Angiogram
Infections[1]	
Epstein-Barr	Blood test
Lyme disease	Blood test
Meningitis	Lumbar puncture
Multiple sclerosis	MRI, lumbar puncture
Mouth	
Abscesses	Dental exam

1. Most infections are accompanied by headache. See text for a complete list.

DISORDER	TEST
Cracked teeth	Dental exam
Eyes	
Eye strain	Eye exam
Glaucoma	Eye exam
Systemic lupus erythematosus (SLE)	Blood test
Giant cell arteritis	Blood test, Biopsy of temporal artery
Polymyalgia rheumatica	Blood test
Mitral valve prolapse	Echocardiogram
Cushing's syndrome	Dexamethasone-suppression test
Head injuries	
Concussion	Depends on severity of injury
Whiplash	

Many neuralgias causing facial pain are beyond the scope of this book. They have distinctive pain patterns and are seldom mistaken for migraine.

I have had a MRI, an echocardiogram, a dental exam, an eye exam, and a variety of blood tests. Because my symptoms did not include a fever, I was not tested for meningitis. All of my tests were negative. It is important to note that you could test positive for one of these conditions and not have all of the symptoms listed in the chapter.

In summary, it would be wise to have a complete physical examination, including a CAT scan or MRI, to rule out headache as a symptom of an underlying disorder. This is especially true if your headaches are new or have changed in their frequency, intensity, or characteristics.

6

Hormones and Migraine

As many as 60 percent of the women prone to migraine find that their headaches intensify just prior to, during, or immediately after menstruation. Decreasing estrogen levels seem to play a role in the migraines experienced during this period. One theory holds that estrogen controls the release of serotonin. As estrogen levels fall, serotonin decreases and vasodilation results.

Anaprox (naproxen), Inderal (propranolol), and various ergotamine preparations are the more common medications used in the treatment of menstrual migraine. However, these drugs, as well as the other medications discussed in chapter 2, have limited success in preventing headaches associated with menstruation. Ponstel (mefenamic acid) is a nonsteroidal anti-inflammatory drug, not discussed in chapter 2, that is used to treat menstrual migraine. Danocrine (danazol), a synthetic androgen, has also been used with some success in the treatment of migraine associated with menstruation. Prophylactic migraine medications are usually begun three days before menses begins and are continued throughout the period of menstruation.

More than 70 percent of female migraine sufferers find that their headaches improve during the second and third trimester of pregnancy only to return after delivery. Some women experience migraines for the first time following delivery. A minority of women who have had migraines all of their lives find that their headaches worsen during pregnancy.

Some researchers feel that high estrogen and progesterone levels during the second and third trimester account for the decrease in migraines. Other researchers stress the correlation between low headache levels and increased production of endorphins during these months. Endorphins are called the body's natural pain killers because of their narcotic-like properties.

Most drugs that treat or prevent migraines cannot be taken by pregnant women for fear they will harm the fetus. One headache authority feels that Demerol (meperidine) is a safe migraine medication that can be taken during pregnancy if it is not taken every day and if daily doses do not exceed 400 mg.[1] Tylenol (acetaminophen) is also considered safe by most physicians. Many feel that aspirin, on the other hand, should be avoided by pregnant women. If you have migraines and are pregnant, check with your doctor before taking any headache medications. Fortunately, headaches usually disappear after the first trimester, and medication will not be needed after that period.

You might think that synthetic estrogen and progesterone added to a woman's natural supply of these hormones would decrease migraines much as an overabundance of hormones decreases headaches during pregnancy. Such is not the case with the birth control pill. Some women experience migraines for the first time while taking "the pill." Fifty percent of migraine sufferers who take oral contraceptives find that their headaches increase in intensity. As can be expected with the serendipity of this disorder, a small number of women find their headaches improve when they take birth control pills.

For most women with pre-existing migraine, headaches occur during the week between cycles when the pill is stopped and hormone levels fall. Women who had migraines for the first time while taking birth control pills do not fall into this pattern. In addition, migraine sufferers, especially those with classic migraine, increase their risk of stroke and other blood vessel disorders when taking oral contraceptives. If you are subject to migraines, birth control pills should be replaced with other forms of contraception.

---

1. Raskin, N.H. (1988): *Headache*. New York: Churchill Livingstone, p. 155.

As estrogen and progesterone decrease during menopause, some women begin to experience migraines for the first time. Almost 50 percent of migraine sufferers find that their headaches worsen when their menstrual cycles stop. Paradoxically, in a minority of women, headaches decrease or stop altogether during menopause. In many cases, estrogen replacement therapy (ERT) tends to intensify pre-existing migraines. However, a small minority of women found that ERT helped their headaches. In these cases, synthetic estrogen was more beneficial than estrogen derived from animal sources.

Three years after beginning menopause, I began to experience daily headaches. I thought that ERT would replicate my pre-menopausal hormonal environment and I would only get migraines during the phase in the monthly cycle when synthetic estrogen was stopped. During the six months I was on ERT, and contrary to all logic, my headaches not only continued on a daily basis, they actually increased in intensity. Perhaps my experience would have been different if I had tried the noncyclic method in which a small amount of estrogen and progesterone is taken each day in the month with no break.

Why does a drop in estrogen cause headaches during menstruation and menopause? One theory, discussed at the beginning of this chapter, stresses the fact that serotonin is controlled by falling estrogen levels. As serotonin levels decline, blood vessels in the brain dilate producing headache.

Why would increased amounts of estrogen due to ERT or the birth control pill cause headaches? Examination of the endometrial tissue of women taking oral contraceptives has shown an increase in monoamine oxidase (MAO). MAO is an enzyme that metabolizes serotonin. Reduced serotonin levels can cause vasodilation and headache.

In summary, it appears that whenever estrogen is either increased synthetically, as in ERT or the contraceptive pill, or decreased dramatically, as in menstruation or menopause, headache often results. Scientific investigation has provided us with little proof as to how altered estrogen levels produce headaches. At this point the connection between estrogen and migraines is purely speculative.

7

Mixed Headaches

Many people experience both migraine and muscle contraction, or tension, headaches. What is the difference between these two types of headache? Muscle contraction headaches are commonly thought to arise from a state of tension in the body. When the body is tense, muscles in the head and neck contract, thus giving rise to pain. Migraine, on the other hand, seems to come from a chemical alteration in the body that leads to dilated blood vessels.

Muscle contraction headaches may be either acute or chronic. Chronic muscle contraction headaches may occur daily or almost daily. In mixed headaches, migraine is superimposed upon, or alternates with, the muscle contraction headache. Sometimes the muscle contraction component of the mixed headache syndrome is, in fact, a rebound headache caused by daily use of analgesics or ergotamine. Over 1000 mg of aspirin or acetaminophen (Tylenol) taken on a daily basis can cause chronic rebound headaches.

Muscle contraction headaches may be experienced as a tight band around the head that can radiate into the neck and shoulders. The pain is usually felt on both sides of the head, whereas the pain in migraine is commonly on one side only. The pain is often dull and constant. It does not pulsate as in a migraine headache. Visual abnormalities and nausea or vomiting do not usually accompany muscle contraction headaches.

Muscle contraction headaches may be a symptom of depression as well as emotional stress. Frustration has been known to trigger a muscle contraction headache. Sometimes these headaches have a purely physical cause, such as sitting hunched over a typewriter or word processor for a long period of time.

Some people may react in a psychologically normal fashion to stressful situations, but their muscles, for reasons unknown to medical science, contract in such a way that headache results. When stressed, all animals, including humans, experience a fight or flight reaction. Muscles contract in preparation for fight or flight. Why in some cases such muscle contraction is accompanied by headache and in other cases it is not is unknown.

In migraine headaches, pain results from the dilation of blood vessels in the brain. In contrast, the pain in muscle contraction headaches is caused by muscles that are in a state of contraction or spasm. Blood vessels have been found to be constricted during headache periods.

Muscle contraction headaches that occur infrequently, say once or twice a month, can usually be treated with aspirin. If stronger medication is needed, Fiorinal tablets or capsules have been successful in eliminating the pain associated with these headaches. Fiorinal, with or without codeine, is composed of aspirin, caffeine, and butalbital, a barbiturate. Butalbital has muscle relaxant properties that make it particularly effective in treating muscle contraction headaches.

I have found exercise to be helpful in eliminating my infrequent muscle contraction headaches. The following three exercises will reduce neck and shoulder tension:

1. Lay on your back on a carpeted floor with your knees flexed and arms at your sides. Raise your shoulders up toward your ears then return to starting position. Repeat ten times.

2. Lay on your back on a carpeted floor with your knees flexed. Alternately raise each arm straight back until the back of your finger tips touch the floor, maintaining a continuous motion. Repeat each cycle fifteen times.

3. Lay on your back on a carpeted floor with knees flexed. Rest hands on your stomach. Turn your head as far to the left as you can. Return to center and then turn your head as far as you can to the right. Repeat each cycle fifteen times or until neck muscles no longer pull.

Wet heat in the form of a damp washcloth on top of a heating pad applied to the back of the neck is another method of reducing the pain of muscle contraction headaches.

If muscle contraction headaches occur frequently, a concerted effort might have to be made to investigate methods of achieving relaxation. In addition, you might want to explore the possibility of taking antidepressant medication. Even if you are not depressed, a small dose of antidepressant medication (perhaps as little as 10 mg) may be helpful in muscle contraction headaches as well as migraine. In difficult cases, a beta blocking drug, such as Inderal, may be combined with the antidepressant.

Antianxiety drugs such as Valium (diazepam), Librium (chlordiazepoxide), or Miltown (meprobamate) are to be avoided since they only treat symptoms and do nothing to help you eliminate the cause of your tension or anxiety. In addition, antianxiety drugs, or tranquilizers, are addicting in that you need increased doses of the drug to be effective, and withdrawal symptoms are experienced if it is stopped abruptly. These drugs have been known to cause rebound headaches in migraine sufferers.

Biofeedback has shown good results in reducing the pain of muscle contraction headaches. The goal of this treatment is to learn to control muscle tension through mental imaging. Biofeedback is discussed in detail in chapter 8. Muscle contraction headaches have also been helped by the relaxation that results from daily meditation, yoga, massage, and exercise.

In summary, if muscle contraction headaches are a chronic condition, methods of reducing tension must be investigated. The possibility of depression should be explored. If muscle contraction headaches are infrequent, a drug such as Fiorinal might be of help. People who get frequent mixed headaches might benefit from antidepressant medication.

8

Biofeedback and Other Alternatives

For centuries, Eastern practitioners have been able to control involuntary body processes with the mind. Anyone who has visited India and watched holy men walking barefoot over burning coals will attest to the possibility of such control. Blood pressure, heart rate, muscle tension, and skin temperature are functions of the autonomic nervous system that can be regulated by mental imagery using a technique known as biofeedback.

Biofeedback teaches thought control over body processes by a system of reinforcement. An electromyographic (EMG) monitor measures muscle tension. A visual or auditory signal indicates when relaxation has achieved a reduction in muscle tension. The desired result is reinforced until muscle tension comes under voluntary control. At this point the EMG monitor is no longer needed. Any technique that reduces muscle tension holds promise in the treatment of muscle contraction headaches.

Vascular, or migraine, headaches have been successfully treated by increasing hand temperature. In this case, a thermistor is taped to the subject's finger to measure skin temperature. This device indicates when thought processes have been successful in increasing hand temperature. The process is reinforced until hand warming can be achieved by voluntary control. As the arteries in the hand dilate, it is believed that those in the head will constrict, thus relieving pain caused by dilated cranial blood vessels. Biofeedback has been most successful in people with classic migraine. In these cases, the headache is aborted during the aura phase before the pain itself is experienced.

One drawback of biofeedback is that the relaxation exercises must be practiced at home every day. The goal of stopping pharmacological treatment, with its unpleasant side effects, is motivation enough for many headache sufferers to try to master this technique. For some people, biofeedback used along with pharmacological therapy allows a reduction in the amount of the drug being used.

Does biofeedback work? Results are mixed. Some researchers have found that relaxation exercises alone are as effective as biofeedback for muscle contraction headaches. In other studies, from 39 to 50 percent of the subjects felt both migraines and muscle contraction headaches had improved. In yet another study, 87 percent experienced improvement. A fewer number of migraine sufferers were able to eradicate their headaches completely when using biofeedback. Nevertheless, any improvement in headache intensity and duration that might allow a reduction in drug use would be of value.

If you want to try biofeedback, it is important that you go to a facility where a professional trained in biofeedback is on staff. If your physician or headache clinic does not offer this modality, ask them to refer you to a pain clinic in your area. Biofeedback is one of the treatment procedures offered by many pain clinics. Be sure the instructor understands that different approaches are used for migraine and muscle contraction headaches. As a migraine sufferer, you will want to learn the hand warming technique. If you have both migraines and muscle contraction headaches, you will also want to learn the muscle tension reduction technique.

Acupuncture is another nondrug modality that has been used to treat migraine. It is an ancient Chinese method of medical treatment in which very fine needles are inserted in the body on specially designated points along what are called meridians. Some practitioners use a battery or electrically powered device to provide electrical stimulation through the needles.

Acupuncture is regarded by many as less effective than biofeedback in migraine treatment. Some improvement might be experienced due to the release of the body's natural painkillers known as endorphins. Studies have shown that over time improvement is temporary. Although acupuncture is a common treatment for headaches in China, Western researchers are less enthusiastic about its long-term benefit for migraine sufferers. Perhaps results in the West are often negative because so many unqualified people are administering this technique. J.N. Blau makes this point in the following quote from a paper by C.A. Vincent and P.H. Richardson.[1]

> To a traditional acupuncturist most of the acupuncture practiced in the west is akin to unqualified person handing out antibiotics at random to sick people. The traditional healer utilizes subtle signs in diagnosis including pulses, the complexion and smell of the patient, whereas trigger points, tender areas, points in the same dermatome as the pain, have little in common with traditional acupuncture other than the insertion of needles.

If you want to try acupuncture, be sure you go to a certified practitioner. Try to find someone trained in the techniques of acupuncture as it has been used over the centuries in traditional Chinese medicine.

Chiropractic therapy offers little help for the migraine sufferer. Chiropractors view disease as stemming from displaced vertebrae that disrupt nerve functioning. Nerve interference can also take place in the muscles and joints. According to chiropractic theory, relieving the pressure on the nerves through manipulation or massage cures certain diseases.

I could find no studies in which chiropractic techniques were shown to abort or prevent migraine headaches. Gentle neck massage may help to relieve muscle contraction headaches. Vigorous manipulation of the neck and spine, however, can be extremely dangerous and should be avoided.

Trager Mentastics is another modality that makes use of the mind-body continuum to relieve pain. The dance-like movements of this approach produce relaxation and a meditative state that serve as a preventative treatment for muscle contraction headaches and for the tension headache component that accompanies migraine in the mixed headache syndrome. Trager Mentastics can be done at home. Trager Psychophysical Integration, on the other hand, is a form of hands-on bodywork done by skilled practitioners.[2] Jan

---

1. Vincent, C.A. and Richardson, P.H. (1986): The evaluation of therapeutic acupuncture: Concepts and methods. *Pain*, 24, 1-13. Reprinted in Blau, J.N., ed. (1987): *Migraine: Clinical and Research Aspects*. Baltimore: The Johns Hopkins University Press.

2. A list of certified Trager practitioners in your area can be obtained by writing to: The Trager Institute, 10 Old Mill Street, Mill Valley, California 94941.

Bennett, Trager practitioner at the Neurologic Centre for Headache and Pain in La Jolla, California, describes this modality as follows:

> With the patient lying on the treatment table the practitioner lifts each body part and with gentle rocking, stretching, compression, and rotation movements encourages the muscles to let go. The practitioner nonverbally supports the patient to experience and incorporate the sensation of muscular lightness and freedom of movement. Trager Psychophysical Integration achieves more lasting results than more traditional methods because the muscle groups are handled in rhythmic, rocking, and stretching motions that prevent both the development of resistance and the return to habitual patterns of tension.

Pain clinics are beginning to realize the importance of body-mind interaction in headache treatment. For example, at the Neurologic Centre for Headache and Pain in La Jolla, California, Trager bodywork is a standard treatment for clients who suffer from tension headaches or migraines with a muscle contraction component. Other modalities used to treat headaches at this facility include medication, psychotherapy, chiropractic treatment, and biofeedback. Chiropractic therapy is used to treat the headache that may result form neck injuries, such as the whiplash injuries associated with automobile accidents. As far as migraine treatment is concerned, Dr. David Hubbard, director of the center, says that they have had the most success with biofeedback. Patients have been found to achieve an 87 percent reduction in the frequency and severity of their migraines in an average of 14 sessions of biofeedback. Trager bodywork is combined with biofeedback if the migraine patient also suffers from tension headaches.

In summary, of the techniques discussed in this chapter, biofeedback holds the most promise for migraine sufferers. If diet and lifestyle changes do not reduce your migraines, biofeedback might be worth exploring. At most, you may be able to abort or prevent your migraines using biofeedback. At the very least, your headaches may be reduced in intensity and duration.

9

Finding the Right Doctor

You have every right to have your headaches taken seriously by your doctor. If he or she implies you are neurotic or tells you your headaches are caused by "nerves," go to another doctor immediately. If he or she wants to treat your migraine headaches with tranquilizers, get another opinion.

Most doctors who specialize in the treatment of migraine are neurologists; however, not all neurologists have the sensitivity, training, or patience to be right for you. You may have to shop around. In the United States, you may want to call the National Headache Foundation in Chicago at 1-800-843-2256 (in Illinois the number is 1-800-523-8858) for a list of physicians in your area who belong to the foundation.

The Migraine Foundation of Canada cannot give the public its membership list of headache specialists. The Canadian Medical Association will only allow this information to be released to physicians. If you live in Canada, ask your doctor to call the Migraine Foundation of Canada in Toronto at (416) 920-4916 for headache specialists in your area.

A list of headache specialists in the United Kingdom can be obtained by calling the Migraine Trust in London at 071-278 2676. In the United Kingdom, a letter of referral is needed from your doctor before an appointment can be made with a specialist.

In Australia your doctor will have to refer you to a headache specialist. Many specialists are associated with the Australian headache clinics listed in Appendix III.

Before going to the doctor, write down a brief description of your headaches and how often you get them. Also include a history of medications you have taken or are taking. Office visits can be hurried, and we sometimes forget important information.

If you do not get migraines very often, the doctor may simply prescribe an anti-inflammatory medication, Midrin, codeine, or some form of ergotamine. If your migraines are frequent, the doctor may start you on a daily dose of a beta blocker or an anti-inflammatory or antidepressant medication. If these medications do not work, a calcium channel blocker or Sansert may be prescribed. Outside of the United States, DHE nasal spray might be prescribed as an abortive agent, and, if daily preventative treatment is necessary, pizotifen might be recommended.

Treatment is usually a case of trial and error when it comes to migraine headaches. If your medication is not effective or you are having side effects, call your doctor. You have the right to be persistent until a medication that relieves your headaches can be found.

Most doctors will ask you to keep a monthly chart on which you will evaluate your migraine on a scale of 1 to 10 while on a particular medication. It is also a good idea to keep a record of your medications and their amounts so you won't repeat ineffective medications years later.

Keeping these kinds of records is part of taking charge of your own health. I have never had a doctor ask me about my diet, for example, even though the headache literature is full of warnings about amine-containing foods. Finding out about the interrelationship of diet, lifestyle, and migraine was up to me. I saw this information as part of becoming an informed consumer. Knowing your medication history is also part of becoming an informed consumer. Finding the right doctor is imperative, but he or she is only one part of your battle to overcome migraine. Total dependence on a doctor will only lead you down the garden path of continued misery.

You might tell a friend, lover, relative, or spouse you have decided to make a renewed effort to conquer your migraines. Ask this person to go to the doctor with you. Keep him or her informed about your medications and changes in your diet or lifestyle. Overcoming migraine is an adventure that can be tedious, and it is nice to have support along the way.

In summary, be patient, but relentless, in your search for a doctor who is knowledgeable and sympathetic. Migraine can be treated if you find the right doctor to work with you to achieve this goal.

10

Basic Steps in Treatment and Prevention

1. Become familiar with the medications used to treat migraine. Review Table 2.1 and the abortive drugs discussed in Appendix I.

2. If you get migraines more than once a week, you might need daily preventative medication. Review the drugs in Table 2.2 and the prophylactic medications discussed in Appendix I.

3. You will have to stop eating amines, nitrites, MSG, sodium benzoate, and the sugar substitute aspartame. You might want to copy Table 3.1 and tape it to a cabinet door in the kitchen as a reminder.

4. Eliminate coffee, tea, caffeine, and all foods containing refined sugar for at least a month to see if your headaches improve.

5. Do not go more than four hours without eating. Have a protein snack before going to bed.

6. Do not get too much or too little sleep.

7. To avoid withdrawal headaches, do not take more than 1000 mg of aspirin or acetaminophen daily and do not take ergotamine every day.

8. Avoid vitamin supplements for a month to see if headaches improve.

9. Have a complete physical examination to rule out headache as a symptom of an underlying disorder.

10. Stop taking birth control pills or estrogen replacement therapy to see if headaches improve.

11. Search until you find a knowledgeable and sensitive doctor who will be diligent in finding medication to abort and/or prevent your migraines.

12. If your medication is not working or has side effects, call your doctor. Be persistent until the right treatment for you is found.

Migraine Portfolio

"Migraine Masterpieces" is the first art competition to be held in the United States on the subject of migraine. Each artist is a migraine sufferer. The work depicts the artist's conception of the debilitating effects of a migraine attack. The competition was sponsored by the National Headache Foundation and Wyeth-Ayerst Laboratories.

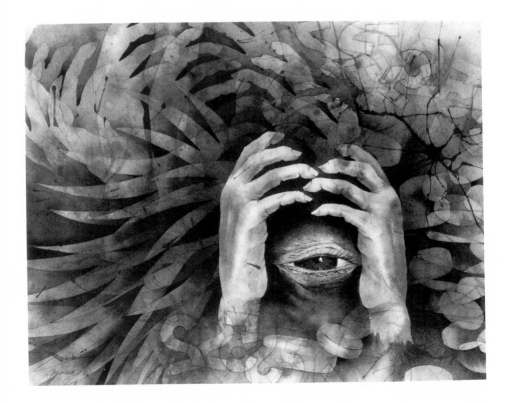

"Violent Passages" by Louise Woodard, Mattydale, NY. The artist focuses on the pain surrounding her eye and the confusion she has with numbers. First prize winner.

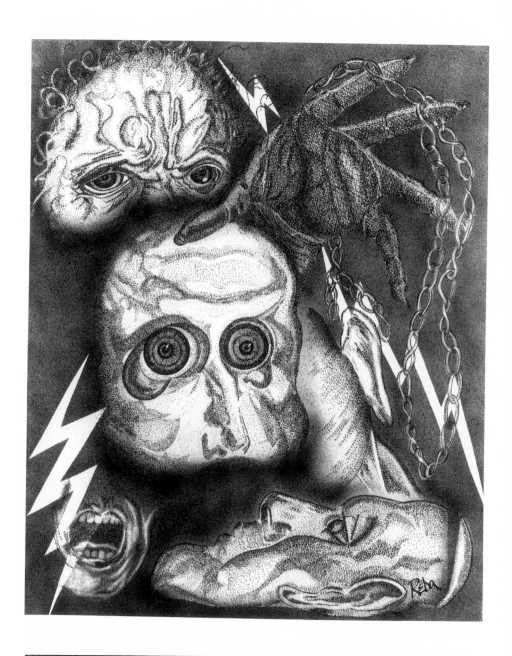

"Nemesis" by Rebecca Whitcanack, Moline, IL. The recurring phantom masks and chains represent the artist's fear of a migraine attack. The bolts of lightning symbolize the pain of migraine. Second prize winner.

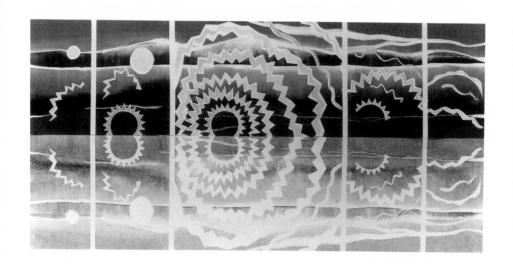

In "Reflections — Five Phases of a Shattered Scape" Carolyn Shaw, San Mateo, CA, portrays the visual experiences of classical migraine.

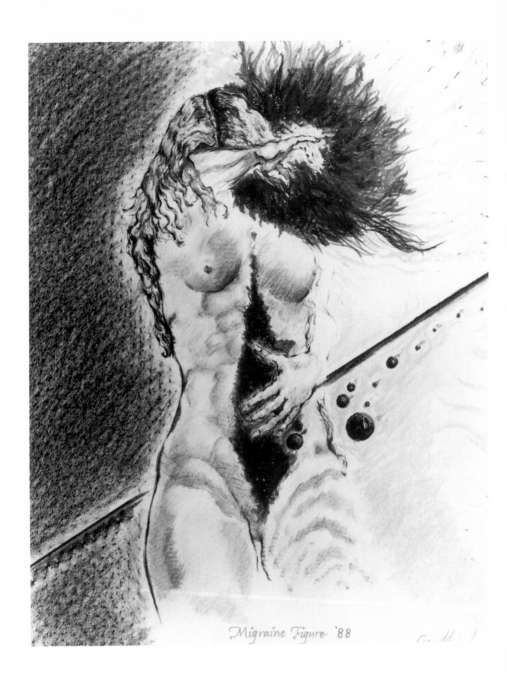

"Migraine Figure" by Constance Mariels, Davis, CA, depicts the exploding head pain and nausea of migraine. Third prize winner.

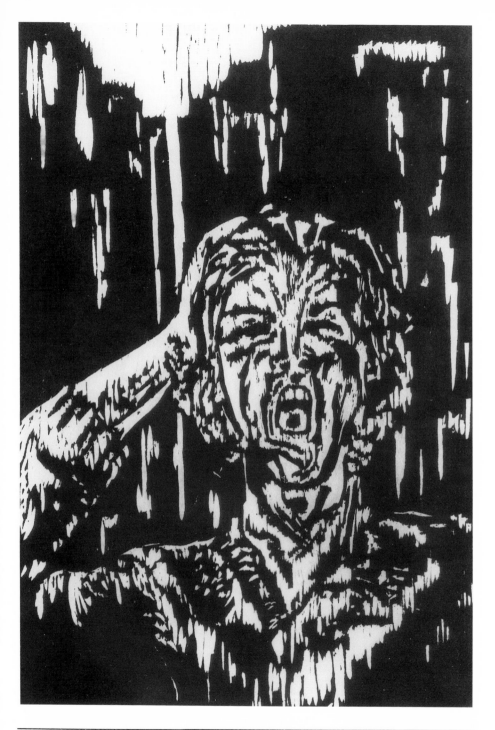

"Frustration, Self-Portrait" by Diane Wilkin, Morrisville, PA, captures the fear and frustration of a migraine attack.

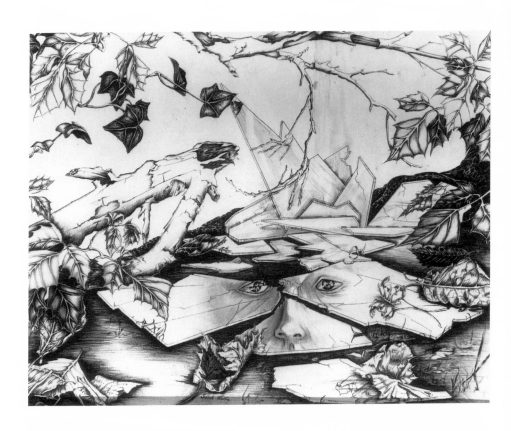

"Migraine" by Sarah Wolfe, Carmel, IN. According to the artist, "Even in the peace of the woods, distorting images, warping sounds — making you someone else — broken and on the ground."

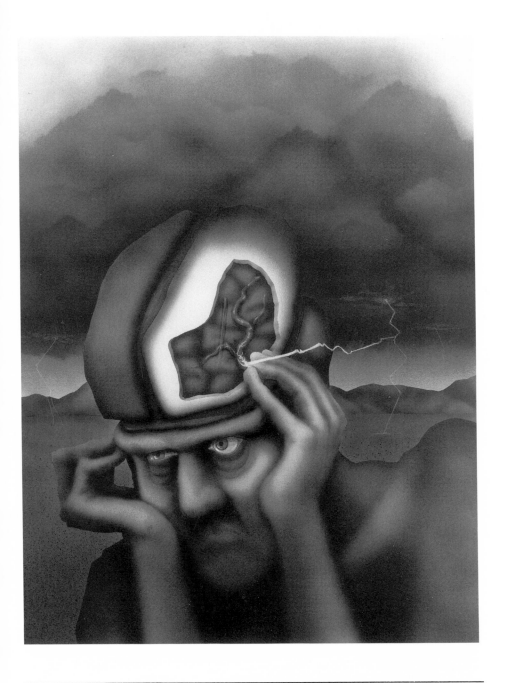

"The Storm Returns" by Thomas Wood, Salt Lake City, UT. In this work we can see how the artist's migraine attacks have depressed and eroded his well-being.

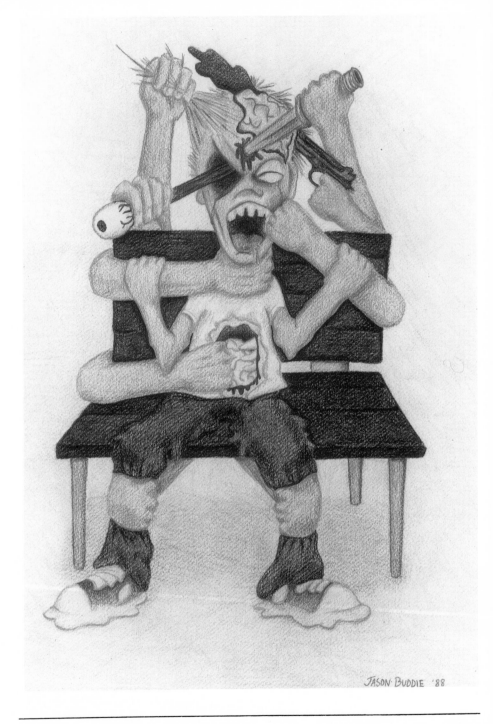

"A Migraine Headache" by Jason Buddie, Brunswick, OH. This young artist captures not only the explosive, wrenching, stabbing, nauseating effects of a migraine attack, but the sense of entrapment within the pain as well.

11

Sharing Information

We can send astronauts to the moon and do heart transplants, but we are still in the dark ages when it comes to migraine. Most medications used to treat migraine, for example, were developed for other applications and were found to help headaches by serendipity. For this reason, all information about migraines is important.

I would like to publish your experience with migraine headaches in the next edition of this book. Please write to me about the nature of your migraines and what you found helpful in treating or preventing them. Letters need only be factual. They do not have to be works of art.

Please state your age and add a note giving me permission to edit and print your letter. If possible, I would appreciate it if you would type your letter, since handwriting is often hard to read. Letters should be sent to me at P.O. Box 422, Village Station, New York, NY 10014.

Your letter will add to the body of information that will one day make it possible for us to conquer this terrible affliction.

Appendix I

Migraine Drugs: Dose, Precautions, Side Effects

Only the most common precautions and side effects are presented. An extremely small percentage of people experience the side effects listed below. For a complete listing check with your doctor.

ABORTIVE MEDICATIONS

Analgesics
Aspirin
Acetaminophen (Tylenol)
Ibuprophen (Advil, Nuprin, Medipren)
Tylenol with codeine

> *Dose:* Follow label for dose. In the case of codeine, take up to 60 mg every 4 hours as needed.[1]
> *Precautions:* Do not combine analgesics. Do not use ibuprophen with diuretics or if you are taking both a beta blocker and a calcium channel blocker.
> *Side effects:* Overuse of aspirin and ibuprophen can cause internal bleeding. Stop taking ibuprophen if you experi-

---

1. *Physicians' Desk Reference (1989):* Oradell, NJ: Medical Economics Co., p. 1244.

ence gastrointestinal bleeding, eye symptoms, rash, water retention, or weight gain.

Comments: To prevent rebound headaches do not exceed 1000 mg of aspirin or Tylenol per day. Codeine should not be taken on a daily basis for any length of time.

Nonsteroidal anti-inflammatory
Anaprox (naproxen sodium)

Dose: 275-825 mg at onset, repeat 275-mg tablet every four hours as needed.[1]

Precautions: Do not use if you are taking Naprosyn, are allergic to aspirin, or have kidney disease. Do not use if you are taking both a beta blocker and a calcium channel blocker. Do not combine with diuretics.

Side effects: Nausea, dizziness, itching skin, fluid retention, headaches, drowsiness, abdominal pain, constipation.

Ergotamine
Cafergot
Wigraine
Medihaler-Ergotamine
Ergomar, Ergostat

Dose: Oral-2 tablets at onset, may repeat 1 tablet every 30 minutes up to 6 per day and 10 per week.[2]
Rectal-1 suppository at onset, may repeat in 1 hour up to 2 per day and 5 per week.[3]
Sublingual-1 tablet at onset, may repeat 1 tablet every 30 minutes up to 3 per day and 5 per week.[4]
Inhalation-1 inhalation every 5 minutes up to 6 per day and 10 per week.[5]

Precautions: Do not take if you have heart disease, high blood pressure, are elderly, have kidney or liver disease,

---

1. Diamond, S. and Millstein, E. (1988): Current concepts of migraine therapy. *Journal of Clinical Pharmacology.* 28: 195.
2. Ibid.
3. Ibid.
4. Ibid.
5. Ibid.

vascular disease, hyperthyroidism, or are taking the antibiotic erythromycin. Do not combine with Midrin or beta blocker.

Side effects: Nausea, diarrhea, pins and needles in hands and feet, elevated blood pressure, leg cramps, abdominal pain, vertigo.

Comments: Daily use can cause rebound headaches. Take with caution during pre-headache aura stage when vessels are constricting. Discontinue use if you experience pins and needles or numbness in hands and feet.

Midrin (isometheptene mucate)

Dose: Take 2 capsules at onset followed by 1 capsule every hour and do not exceed 5 per day or 15 per week.[1]

Precautions: Do not take if you have heart disease, glaucoma, peripheral vascular disease, high blood pressure, severe kidney disease, liver disease, or are taking a MAO inhibitor. Do not combine with ergotamine or beta blockers.

Side effects: Drowsiness, lightheadedness.

Beta blocker

Inderal (propranolol)

Dose: 10-80 mg per day.[2]

Precautions: Contraindications include heart failure, slowed heart rate, very low blood pressure, breathing difficulties, asthma, severe diabetes or hypoglycemia. Do not combine with a MAO inhibitor. Use with caution if you are combining this drug with a calcium channel blocker. Do not use with Tagamet or ergotamine.

Side effects: Fatigue, nausea, depression, lightheadedness, constipation, insomnia, dizziness, diarrhea, vivid dreams, lethargy, breathlessness.

---

1. Ibid.
2. Peatfield, R. (1986): *Headache*, New York: Springer-Verlag, p.122.

Caffeine
NoDoz

      Dose: 100 to 200 mg per day.
  Comment: Do not exceed dose by combining with coffee, tea, or soft drinks.

NAUSEA
Reglan (metoclopramide)

      Dose: One 10 mg dose daily.[1]
 Precautions: To prevent additive sedative effects do not combine with alcohol, sedatives, hypnotics, tranquilizers, or narcotics. Do not take if using a MAO inhibitor.
 Side effects: Fatigue, drowsiness, restlessness, anxiety. Dystonic reactions (involuntary movements of limbs and facial grimacing) occur in approximately 1 out of 500 patients treated with 30-40 mg/day.[2]

PROPHYLACTIC MEDICATIONS

Beta blockers
Inderal (propranolol)
Corgard (nadolol)
Blocadren (timolol)

      Dose: Inderal: Begin at 80 mg per day and maintain at 160-240 mg per day.[3]
  Corgard: Begin at 40 mg once daily and maintain at 40-60 mg once daily.[4]
  Blocadren: 10-20 mg twice daily.[5]
 Precautions: Contraindications include heart failure, slowed heart rate, asthma, low blood pressure, severe diabetes, hypoglycemia, or breathing problems. Do not combine with a MAO inhibitor. Use with caution if

---

1. Ibid., p. 116.
2. *Physicians' Desk Reference,* op. cit., p. 1704.
3. Diamond and Millstein, op. cit., p. 196.
4. Ibid.
5. Ibid.

you are combining this drug with a calcium channel blocker. Do not use with Tagamet or ergotamine.

Side effects: Dizziness, nausea, depression, lethargy, vivid dreaming, diarrhea or constipation, insomnia, fatigue, breathlessness.

Comment: Discontinue use of drug gradually, not suddenly.

Ergotamine
Bellergal
Bellergal-S

Dose: Bellergal: 1 tablet 4 times a day.[1]
Bellergal-S: 1 tablet 2 times a day.[2]

Precautions: Do not take if you have blood vessel disease, high blood pressure, kidney or liver disease, heart disease, glaucoma, asthma. Do not use with Midrin or beta blocker.

Side effects: Blurred vision, drowsiness, dry mouth, palpitations, urinary retention, flushing, pins and needles in limbs.

Comment: Report numbness or tingling in extremities to doctor.

Antidepressants
Elavil (amitriptyline)
Sinequan (doxepin)

Dose: Elavil: 10-175 mg once daily.[3]
Sinequan: 10-150 mg once daily.[4]

Precautions: Do not use if you have heart disease, epilepsy, glaucoma, or are taking a MAO inhibitor. Do not combine with thioridazine (Mellaril). Check with doctor about using Tagamet or drinking alcohol with these drugs.

Side effects: Drowsiness, dry mouth, blurred vision, dizziness, sedation, tingling in fingers, increased dreaming, constipation, urine retention, weight gain, palpitations, lowered blood pressure.

---

1.   Ibid.
2.   Ibid.
3.   Raskin, N.H. (1988): *Headache*. New York: Churchill Livingstone, p. 182.
4.   Diamond and Millstein, op. cit., p. 196.

Comment: Taper off if taking more than minimum dose.

Sansert (methysergide)

Dose: 2 mg three times a day.[1]

Precautions: Do not take if you have vascular disease, heart disease, high blood pressure, lung, kidney, or liver disease.

Side effects: Increased appetite, constipation, insomnia or drowsiness, dizziness, hallucinations, chest and abdominal pain, numbness in limbs, disturbance of balance, fibrosis (scar tissue that forms in heart, lungs, or abdomen), diarrhea, hair loss, weight gain, edema, sweating, nausea.

Comments: Take test dose of one-half tablet to see if immediate side effects occur. Stop treatment one month out of four to prevent fibrotic side effects. Report pain, coldness, or numbness in limbs, chest pain, leg cramps, abdominal pain to your doctor.

Calcium channel blockers

Isoptin (verapamil)
Procardia (nifedipine)

Dose: Isoptin: 80-160 mg three times a day.[2]
Procardia: 10-30 mg three times a day.[3]

Precautions: Take with caution if you have liver or kidney disease. Contraindicated in certain kinds of heart disease. Use with caution if combining with a beta blocker. Do not use with the antihistamine Seldane. Do not combine with calciferol or calcium adipinate.

Side effects: Dizziness, edema, constipation, nausea, fatigue, headache, lightheadedness.

Comment: These drugs cause vasodilation and should only be taken when blood vessels are at rest. They should not be taken during the headache phase when the blood vessels are dilated.

---

1.   Ibid.
2.   Ibid.
3.   Ibid.

Appendix II

The Physiology of Migraine: A Recapitulation

In spite of the many theories about migraine, most researchers agree that amines play a role in the development of headache. Some amines, such as serotonin, are made in the body. Other amines are found in the foods we eat. Amines serve many functions, but the one we are most concerned with is their influence on the size of the blood vessels in the brain.

When serotonin is released blood vessels constrict. As serotonin levels fall, the blood vessels dilate, causing pain in the surrounding nerves. What causes serotonin to be released? An increase in estrogen triggers an increase in serotonin. This may be why a birth control pill containing estrogen produces headaches in some women. Conversely, a drop in estrogen levels during menstruation produces a decrease in serotonin, thus triggering vasodilation and headache directly. Stress can also alter serotonin levels. The low blood sugar that results from not eating regularly is another influence on serotonin levels. The amines in the foods we eat cannot be metabolized properly by some people. High levels of these amines trigger a chain reaction that results in vasodilation.

Medications taken once a headache has begun, such as Midrin or ergotamine, constrict the already dilated blood vessels, thus eliminating pain. Other abortive medications, such as aspirin or codeine, simply kill our awareness of the pain without reducing the size of the blood vessels.

Some preventative medications, such as the antidepressants, alter the level of serotonin by binding onto serotonin receptors in the brain. By interfering with the entry of calcium into the cells, the calcium channel blockers decrease serotonin release, inhibit vaso-constriction, and dilate cerebral arteries. These medications should be taken only when the cerebral arteries are in a state of rest. If you were to take a calcium channel blocker once a headache is underway, you would be adding dilation to dilation and the pain would be tremendous.

Even without medication you do have some control over your migraine headaches. By eating regularly, eliminating foods containing amines, and avoiding synthetic estrogen, the vasodilation associated with migraine can be prevented.

Appendix III

Headache Clinics

Please be aware that the treatment policies of the headache clinics listed below will differ. A clinic directed by a psychiatrist will be more inclined to emphasize biofeedback and other nonmedication modalities. A clinic directed by a neurologist will tend to follow a more traditional medical model. In some clinics, as the eclectic approach becomes more popular, these differences will no longer apply.

UNITED STATES

Arizona
Headache Clinic of the Southwest
1402 North Miller Road
Suite F5
Scottsdale, AZ 85257
(602) 941-5353

California
California Medical Clinic
for Headache
16542 Ventura Boulevard
Encino, CA 91436
(818) 986-4248

Headache Treatment Center of
Orange County
14111 Newport Avenue
Tustin, CA 92680
(714) 832-2505

Neurologic Centre for
Headache and Pain
4150 Regents Park Row
Suite 255
La Jolla, CA 92037
(619) 558-4688

The San Francisco Headache
Clinic
909 Hyde Street
Suite 230
San Francisco, CA 94109
(415) 673-4600

Scripps Clinic and Research Foundation
10666 North Torrey Pines Road
La Jolla, CA 92037
(619) 455-9100

Colorado

Colorado Neurology and
Headache Center
1155 East 18 Avenue
Denver, CO 80218
(303) 839-9900

Headache Clinic of Denver
1355 South Colorado Boulevard
Denver, CO 80222
(303) 759-2220

Connecticut

The New England Center for Headache
40 East Putnam Avenue
Cos Cob, CT 06807
(203) 968-1799

Florida

Headache Management
Center
1925 Mizell Avenue
Suite 100
Winter Park, FL 32792
(407) 628-2905

Headache Management and
Neurology
5500 North Davis Highway
Pensacola, FL 32503
(904) 474-0740

Illinois

Diamond Headache Clinic
5252 North Western Avenue
Chicago, IL 60625
(312) 878-5558

Indiana
Tri-State Headache and Pain Management Associates
801 St. Mary's Drive
Suite 302
Evansville, IN 47715
(812) 473-4394

Kansas
Headache Clinic
Department of Neurology
University of Kansas Medical Center
39th and Rainbow Boulevard
Kansas City, KS 66103
(913) 588-6985

Maryland
Baltimore Headache Institute
11 East Chase Street
Suite 1A
Baltimore, MD 21202
(301) 547-0200

Massachusetts
John R. Graham Headache Centre
Faulkner Hospital
Allendale at Centre Street
Jamaica Plain, MA 02130
(617) 522-6969

Michigan

Department of Neurology
Henry Ford Hospital
2799 West Grand Boulevard
Detroit, MI 48202
(313) 876-2600

Michigan Headache and
Neurological Institute
3120 Professional Drive
Ann Arbor, MI 48104
(313) 973-1155

Minnesota
Headache Institute of Minnesota
2545 Chicago Avenue
Suite G-10
Minneapolis, MN 55404
(612) 870-8066

New York

The Downstate Headache
Center
132 Atlantic Avenue
Brooklyn, NY 11201
(718) 935-9666

Elkind Headache Clinic
20 Archer Avenue
Mt. Vernon, NY 10550
(914) 667-2230

Headache Clinic
Mount Sinai Medical Center
1 Gustave Levy Place
New York, NY 10029
(212) 241-7691

Headache Unit
Montefiore Medical Center
111 East 210 Street
Bronx, NY 10467
(212) 920-4636

Ohio

Headache Department
Cleveland Clinic Foundation
9500 Euclid Avenue
Cleveland, OH 44106
(216) 444-5654

Texas

Dallas Headache Clinic
8226 Douglas Avenue
Suite 325
Douglas Plaza
Dallas, TX 75225
(214) 692-7011

Houston Headache Clinic
1213 Hermann Drive
Houston, TX 77004
(713) 528-1916

CANADA

Ask your doctor to call the Migraine Foundation of Canada in Toronto at (416) 920-4916 for headache clinics in your area. This listing is not available to the public.

UNITED KINGDOM

Admission to the following clinics is dependent upon a referral from your doctor.

England

The City of London
Migraine Clinic
22 Charterhouse Square
London EC1M 6DX
(01) 251-3322

Hull Royal Infirmary
Anlaby Road
Hull HU3 2J2
(0482) 28541

King's College Hospital
Denmark Hill
London SE5 9RS
(01) 274 6222

Royal Infirmary
Preston
Lancashire PR1 6PS
(0772) 716565

The Princess Margaret Migraine Clinic
Charing Cross Hospital
Fulham Palace Road
London W6 8RF
(01) 471 7833

Scotland

Migraine Clinic
Western General Hospital
Crewe Road
Edinburgh EH4 2XU
(031) 332 2525

AUSTRALIA

Please obtain a referral letter from your doctor before making an appointment.

New South Wales

Department of Neurology
Royal North Shore Hospital
Pacific Highway
St. Leonards
New South Wales 2065
(2) 438-7111

Neurology Clinic
Prince Henry Hospital
Anzac Parade
Little Bay
New South Wales 2036
(2) 661-0111

Queensland
Headache Clinic
Royal Brisbane Hospital
Herston Road
Herston
QLD 4006
(7) 253-8111

South Australia

Headache and Pain Clinic
Queen Elizabeth Hospital
Woodville Road
Woodville
SA 5011
(8) 45-0222

Neurology Clinic
Flinders Medical Centre
South Road
Bedford Park
SA 5042
(8) 275-9911

Appendix IV

Migraine Associations

National Headache Foundation
5252 North Western Avenue
Chicago, IL 60625
In Illinois 1-800-523-8858
Outside Illinois 1-800-843-2256

Migraine Foundation of Canada
390 Brunswick Avenue
Toronto, Ontario M5R 224
Canada
(416)920-4916

The Migraine Trust
45 Great Ormond Street
London WC1N 3HD
England
071-278 2676

Annotated Bibliography

Blau, J.N., ed. (1987): *Migraine: Clinical and Research Aspects*. Baltimore: The Johns Hopkins University Press.

A comprehensive medical textbook on migraine. Each chapter is written by a noted authority in the field. Various theories on the causes of migraine, drug therapy, and nonpharmacological treatments are some of the subjects explored.

Braunwald, E.; Isselbacher, K.J.; Petersdorf, R.G.; Wilson, J.D.; Martin, J.B.; and Fauci, A.S., eds. (1987): *Harrison's Principles of Internal Medicine*. New York: McGraw-Hill.

One of the major texts on internal medicine for physicians. Contains a discussion of disorders that may be accompanied by headache.

Brody, J.E. (1988, October 11): Studies unmask origins of brutal migraines. *The New York Times*, pp. C1, C10.

The role of serotonin in the development of migraine is discussed.

Dalessio, D.J., ed. (1987): *Wolff's Headache and Other Head Pain*. New York: Oxford University Press.

A revised and updated edition of a classic textbook on headaches. Two chapters are specifically devoted to migraine.

Diamond, S., ed. (1990): *Migraine Headache Prevention and Management*. New York and Basel: Marcel Dekker.

A comprehensive text for physicians. Chapters are written by well-known headache authorities. Recommended for the reader who wishes to explore in depth the science of migraine treatment and prevention.

Diamond, S. and Millstein, E. (1988): Current concepts of migraine therapy. *J. Clin. Pharmacol.* 28: 193-199.

This article contains a thorough discussion of the abortive and prophylactic drugs currently used to treat migraine.

Diener, H.C. and Wilkinson, M., eds. (1988): *Drug-Induced Headache.* New York: Springer-Verlag.

Explores how headaches may be caused by the chronic use of some headache medications.

Ferrari, M.D. and Lataste, X., eds. (1989): *Migraine and Other Headaches.* Carnforth, Lancs. and Park Ridge, N.J.: The Parthenon Publishing Group.

The section on pharmacological treatments is particularly helpful to the migraine sufferer who wishes to investigate the research aspects of drug therapies.

Glover, V. and Sandler, M. (1990): New developments in the biochemistry of migraine—focus on 5-HT. *Headache Quarterly: Current Treatment and Research* 1: 174-176.

The association between serotonin (5-HT), selected medications, and migraine is explored.

Hancock, K. (1986): *Feverfew: Your Headache May Be Over.* New Canaan, Conn.: Keats Publishing.

Written for the general public with many testimonials by people who have been helped by feverfew.

Levine, H.W. (1988-1989): Special report: International congress presents new therapy for migraine sufferers. *National Headache Foundation Newsletter* 67: 1-3.

Glaxo's new drug, GR 43175, now undergoing clinical trials, is discussed.

Low, R. (1987): *Migraine: The Breakthrough Study that Explains what Causes it and How it Can Be Completely Prevented through Diet.* New York: Henry Holt.

Explores the role of sugar as a migraine trigger.

Medina, J.L. and Diamond, S. (1978): The role of diet in migraine. *Headache* 18: 31-34.

Foods that contain the vasodilator tyramine, and their role as migraine triggers are presented.

Peatfield, R. (1986): *Headache*. New York: Springer-Verlag.

A concise medical textbook written for physicians. The chapters on the clinical aspects of migraine, precipitating causes, the treatment of the acute attack, and preventative measures would be of interest to migraine sufferers.

Physicians' Desk Reference (1989): E.R. Barnhart, publisher. Oradell, N.J.: Medical Economics Co.

The dose, precautions, contraindications, and adverse reactions of all prescription medications available in the United States are discussed in this standard reference.

Raskin, N.H. (1988): *Headache*. New York: Churchill Livingstone.

An excellent medical textbook by a noted headache authority. The sections on precipitating factors and pharmacological treatment are especially pertinent.

Rose, F.C., ed. (1988): *The Management of Headache*. New York: Raven Press.

A research-oriented medical text based on a series of lectures organized by the Migraine Trust and presented to physicians at the Charing Cross Hospital and Westminster Medical School.

Sacks, O. (1985): *Migraine: Understanding a Common Disorder*. Berkeley and Los Angeles: University of California Press.

Contains a comprehensive description of common migraine, classical migraine, and migraine equivalents. Factors that may precipitate a migraine attack are explored. The section on treatment is very weak. This book was written for the general public and is available in paperback.

Sandweiss, J. (1989): Biofeedback in the treatment of headaches. *National Headache Foundation Newsletter* 70: 1-3.

The author discusses ways biofeedback can be used to treat tension headaches and migraine.

Steinmetzer, R.V. (1989): Combination drug treatment for headaches. *National Headache Foundation Newsletter* 68: 2-3.

The actions and interactions of drugs commonly used to treat headaches are presented.

Glossary

Abortive medication Medication that is used to terminate a migraine headache once it has begun.

Acetaminophen A popular analgesic. Most commonly known by the brand name Tylenol.

Acupuncture An ancient Chinese method of relieving pain or curing disease by inserting needles into especially designated points in the body.

Amines Substances found in food or made in the body that serve many functions, including regulating mood and the diameter of the blood vessels.

Analgesics Drugs used to reduce the awareness of pain.

Androgen Male sex hormone. The synthetic form of this hormone has been used to treat menstrual migraine.

Antidepressants Drugs used to alter mood (in depression) and blood vessel diameter (in migraine) because of their ability to control the level of amines in the body.

Antiemetic drugs Drugs that are used to relieve nausea and vomiting.

Atypical migraine Gastrointestinal distress, visual abnormalities, or other symptoms associated with migraine may be present unaccompanied by

	noticeable head pain. Also called migraine equivalents.
Aura	Symptoms that precede the headache phase in classic migraine.
Beta blockers	A class of drugs used to treat people with heart problems. A secondary benefit of these drugs was discovered when heart patients found that their migraine headaches also improved.
Biofeedback	A method by which people are taught to become aware of their heart rate, blood pressure, muscle tension, and skin temperature in order to consciously control these processes.
Calcium channel blockers	Drugs that prevent constriction of the blood vessels by interfering with the entry of calcium into the cells.
Chiropractic therapy	A method of manipulation used to treat headaches resulting from cervical spine disorders.
Classic migraine	Visual abnormalities, vertigo, tingling, numbness, confusion, nausea, mood changes, or speech disturbances are experienced before the onset of the headache phase.
Common migraine	No specific symptoms are experienced prior to the headache itself.
Ergotamine	A fungus that grows on rye that has the ability to constrict dilated blood vessels.
Estrogen	A female sex hormone. Decreasing levels just before menstruation trigger migraine in some women.
Hypoglycemia	An abnormally low concentration of sugar in the blood causing such symptoms as headache, sweating, and light-headedness.
Ibuprophen	An analgesic that has anti-inflammatory properties if taken in a large enough dose. Brand names include Nuprin, Medipren, and Advil.
Menstrual migraine	Migraine headaches that occur prior to or during menstruation.

Migraine	A headache that is often throbbing in nature and usually confined to one side of the head. Visual disturbances, nausea, and other symptoms may precede or accompany the headache. The pain of the headache phase is caused by dilated blood vessels.
Migraine triggers	Dietary, environmental, chemical, or hormonal substances, as well as emotional factors, that cause a reaction in the body resulting in vasodilation and headache.
Muscle contraction headache	A dull, constant pain that may feel like a tight band around the head. The cause of the headache is most often attributed to such emotional factors as stress, frustration, anxiety, or depression. Also referred to as a tension headache.
Neurotransmitter	Chemical released at the junction of two nerve cells that allows or prevents the passing of electrical impulses from one nerve cell to another.
Nonsteroidal anti-inflammatories	These drugs inhibit platelet aggregation which has been linked to the release and destruction of serotonin. They also inhibit certain vasodilators known as prostaglandins.
Octopamine	A vasoactive amine found in citrus that can trigger a migraine in susceptible individuals.
Phenylethylamine	An amine found in chocolate and other foods that can trigger a headache in susceptible people because of its vasoactive properties.
Progesterone	A female sex hormone. Levels of the hormone decrease just before the onset of menstruation.
Prophylactic medication	A medication that is taken daily to prevent migraine headaches from occurring.
Rebound headache	A headache caused by the chronic overuse of such chemical agents as ergotamine, caffeine, and analgesics. See *Withdrawal symptoms*
Serotonin	An amine found throughout the human body. Levels of this amine increase prior to a

migraine attack and decrease once the headache begins.

Sinus headache
When the sinuses cannot drain properly because of infection or allergy a headache similar to migraine may result.

Status migrainosus
A prolonged migraine attack in which the headache may change in intensity, but never really disappears.

Trager Mentastics
An excercise using dance-like movements to produce a relaxed, meditative state. Used as preventative treatment for the muscle contraction component of the mixed headache syndrome.

Trager psycho-physical integration
A modality used to reduce tension in which the practitioner teaches the patient to use his or her muscles in a less restricted manner.

Tryptophan
An amino acid found in turkey and other foods that is a precursor to the synthesis of serotonin.

Tyramine
An amine found in cheese and many other foods that produces vasodilation and migraine in susceptible individuals.

Vasoconstriction
Describes blood vessels that have decreased in diameter.

Vasodilation
Describes blood vessels that have increased in diameter.

Withdrawal symptoms
Symptoms caused by the abrupt stopping of a drug to which one has become habituated. More of the drug is then taken to relieve the symptoms caused by the cessation.

Index

About the Author

Betsy H. Wyckoff has been a college textbook development editor in medicine, the social sciences, and the humanities for many years. At present, she is a freelance writer. She is an avid art collector and photographer in her spare time.

She majored in premed and English literature as an undergraduate student. More recently, she obtained an M.A. degree in counseling psychology.

Ms. Wyckoff lives in New York City.